The Efficient Physician

7 Guiding Principles for a Tech-Savvy Practice

SECOND EDITION

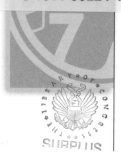

Sherry Anderson Delio
MPA, HSA, FACMPE

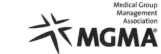
Medical Group
Management
Association

MGMA®

Medical Group Management Association
104 Inverness Terrace East
Englewood, CO 80112-5306
877.275.6462
Web site: www.mgma.com

PUBLISHER'S CATALOGING-IN-PUBLICATION DATA

Delio. Sherry Anderson.
　　The Efficient Physician, 2nd Ed.: 7 Guiding Principles for a Tech-Savvy Practice / Sherry Anderson Delio.
　　p. 128 ; cm.
　　Includes bibliographical references and index.
　　ISBN 1-56829-233-3
　　1. Medical offices – Management. 2. Group medical practice – Management. 3. Medical offices – Automation. 4. Information storage and retrieval systems—Medical care. 5. Professional Practice – organization & administration.

I. Title: The Efficient Physician, 2nd Ed. II. Delio, Sherry A. III. Title.
R858.D353 2005
658'.059—dc22   2005926268

Item #6341

Printed in the United States of America
10 9 8 7 6 5 4 3 2

DEDICATION

To my daughter Angie,
whose courage inspires me daily.

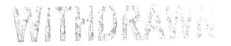

Contents

	About the Author	vii
	Preface	ix
	Acknowledgments	xi
1	Introduction	1
2	A Chaotic Medical Practice	5
3	The 7 Guiding Principles	11
4	Best Value in Town	17
5	Seeing Your Practice through Your Patients' Eyes	21
6	**PRINCIPLE I:** Real-time Work	29
7	**PRINCIPLE II:** Making a Time Commitment	31
8	**PRINCIPLE III:** Balancing Workloads	43
9	**PRINCIPLE IV:** Decreasing Unnecessary Variation	49
10	**PRINCIPLE V:** Distributing Tasks Appropriately	67
11	**PRINCIPLE VI:** Creating an Interdependent Team	75
12	**PRINCIPLE VII:** Allocating Resources by Volume of Work	85
13	A Smooth Operation	89
14	A Tech-Savvy Practice	95
15	Tying It All Together	103
	Glossary	111
	Index	115

About the Author

Sherry Anderson Delio, MPA, HSA, FACMPE, President of Delio Consulting, is a registered nurse who has been working as a group management administrator and a practice management consultant since 1984. She holds a master's degree in public administration with an emphasis in health services administration from the University of San Francisco. She also became a Fellow of the American College of Medical Practice Executives in 2004.

Delio, a member of both MGMA and ACMPE, uses work measurement methodologies to improve workflow and to help physicians understand how to maximize their time and maintain a viable practice while balancing their personal life. Sherry began her work in a hospital setting, moved to group practice, then academic practices, and now is focusing her work on rural medicine.

Sherry has worked on three Institute of Healthcare Improvement (IHI) initiatives related to access and wait-time initiatives – one as a participant and two as faculty. She also speaks nationally on practice improvement issues.

In addition, Sherry is the co-author of the first edition of *The Making of an Efficient Physician*, and author of *The Perfect Practice for an Efficient Physician*.

Preface

With today's ultra-competitive marketing and recruitment strategies (for patients, staff and physicians!), every medical practice must become more efficient to survive and thrive. Inefficient practices have lower levels of patient satisfaction and eventually lose patients and revenue to better-performing practices. These disorganized practices aren't great places to work, either – low staff and physician morale also negatively affect practice operations. In this new edition of the MGMA classic, *The Making of an Efficient Physician*, the author addresses medical practice chaos with common sense and high-tech strategies, demonstrating that efficient systems and appropriate technology are the keys to survival and success.

This new edition identifies where problems generally exist, how to find them, and how to implement change in nearly any size practice. Author Sherry Delio illustrates through real-life examples what occurs in an unsystematic practice (do you recognize anyone in this scenario?) and how to implement changes to create a smooth-running medical office that surprises and delights its patients. She also introduces the electronic health record and explains how this technology streamlines practices by providing physicians, staff and patients with quick access to information and scheduling options.

The book not only updates the author's proven guidelines for revamping or setting up core practice systems, it also explains the importance of working in real time

– her newest Guiding Principle for an efficient practice. Each chapter explores how to achieve success by following each of the 7 Guiding Principles:

1. **Real-time Work** – Do today's work today.

2. **Time Commitment** – Commit time to yourself, your patients and your practice.

3. **Balanced Workloads** – Take control of your physician and patient schedules.

4. **Decreased Variations** – Standardize and eliminate unnecessary variations.

5. **Appropriate Task Distribution** – Delegate tasks correctly and wisely.

6. **Interdependent Teamwork** – Create a team that really works together.

7. **Resource Allocation** – Watch your volume and adjust resources correctly.

If you are a physician, office manager, health care executive, nurse, nonphysician provider or medical student, you will learn something new in this book. It is succinct, easy-to-read, straight-to-the-point and complete with essential and easy-to-implement tips that identify weak areas and suggest how to replace them with patient-focused systems. You will obtain simple, proven strategies that net results: a practice with improved efficiency, enhanced technology, and increased profitability.

Acknowledgments

I would like to thank all the wonderful physicians, nurses and other staff members I have been fortunate to work with over the past 20 years. They continually teach me the importance of staying true to our mission of improving health care – one day at a time.

I would also like to thank the true leaders in health care improvement that never lose site of a health care system that meets the intent of our constitution – to care for the general welfare of all.

It is my belief that if the health care community will unite, we can solve the health care problems we face today. However, if the private sector does not step up, the government will be forced to step in.

Of course, I would like to thank my husband Tony, who has to put up with the hours I spend at the computer. I would like to thank my adult children, Darin, Monica and Angie for making my life complete.

A special thanks goes to the support of the Medical Group Management Association (MGMA) and especially Cyndy Mitchell, my editor.

| # Introduction

CELL PHONES, PERSONAL DIGITAL ASSISTANTS, E-MAIL and the Internet – technology runs our world. It is constantly improving communication and organization tools that help us use our time more efficiently. Today, we can access information instantly on the Internet; we can carry a small computer in a pocket to see our schedule, send e-mail messages and update documents; and we can send text messages and take photos with our cell phones.

How can a physician or medical practice harness current and emerging technologies to help improve practice efficiency, and increase patient satisfaction and workplace fulfillment?

This book shows you what happens in a disorganized, chaotic practice, and presents practice management principles to implement effective and efficient systems for superior practice management. We also introduce you to an emerging technology – the electronic health record (EHR) and show how, when married with efficient operating systems, the EHR can enhance your practice service to exceed both patient and practice expectations.

Core practice systems

The following chapters present overall Guiding Principles and delineate clear proactive steps to help you develop a more efficient practice. When you have finished the book, you will have completed a crash course in the skills that will set your practice up for continued success. Quite simply, you will learn to eliminate wasted time and effort, to work efficiently and to create an environment in which physicians can care for more patients with less stress.

We provide sample documents for you to use in your practice as you identify areas that need better systems and to use after you've streamlined processes.

We show how an EHR provides a document tool that monitors patient health status over time (instead of just a chronological list of episodic activities); and how the EHR allows you to share information with patients and encourage shared responsibility for care. This contributes to genuine value – appropriate and timely care, quality outcomes, excellent service and reasonable prices – offered to your patients.

By using the key management principles in this book, you can immediately enhance patient care by improving the operational systems that support the patient-physician interaction.

Balance your life

In years of consulting with physicians, one of the most common laments we hear is, "If I could only spend more time taking care of patients and less time on paperwork, I would be happy." Balancing work and personal time can be a difficult goal, but if you implement and follow the guidelines in this book, you can achieve it. The book shows managers how to design operations based on solid systems, how to use open communication and time-efficient protocols with a general concern for patient, physician and staff satisfaction, and how to augment your practice using the EHR. As a result, physicians can care for additional patients in a more orderly, relaxed way. The practice also will gain a reputation among patients, staff and other physicians as being a place of true value – the key competitive advantage today.

The electronic health record (EHR) system

What is it? Do I need it? How will it change my practice? Will it help my practice? We hear these questions every day. Moving toward an EHR is a major decision in medical practices today, yet few understand the fundamental changes the EHR will make to their practice.

Access to information, improved documentation and patient safety issues are motivating more and more practices to implement an EHR. The Guiding Principles set forth in the following chapters will give you a road map for developing an efficient practice before you take it to the next level by implementing an EHR. By teaming an EHR with the practice management principles stated in this book, you can have the practice you have always wanted – information at your fingertips, early identification of adverse trends, early inter-vention detection, instant patient education materials, complete medical records, and control over your time and practice.

Marketplace competition

Today's marketplace competition for patients is ever increasing. Physicians must embrace tools that will give them the edge over competitors. If you are ready to revamp your practice, set up a new practice or just learn something new, let's get started!

CHAPTER 2

A Chaotic Medical Practice

LACK OF A CLEAR UNDERSTANDING about how physicians practice often results in operating systems that inhibit rather than enhance physician productivity and customer service. Well-designed processes are essential in an efficient, effective medical practice.

The following fictitious case illustrates behavior witnessed during physician workflow studies of hundreds of physician practices in different regions around the United States. Few practices are as chaotic as Dr. Frazzle's, but many of these problems occur in numerous practices. Inefficient systems compromise quality patient care. When physicians don't have the information they need when they need it, chaos reigns and patient satisfaction plummets.

Let's visit Dr. Frazzle's practice and see how well-intentioned activities can eat away at a physician's time and be misinterpreted by the patient. Then remember this scenario when you read Chapter 13 to learn how Dr. Frazzle could have handled this day in a more efficient, satisfying manner – for himself, his staff and his patient.

Welcome to Dr. Frazzle's practice

Ms. Ann Ackney knew she needed a follow-up appointment. She did not hear from the doctor's office as promised, so she decided to call and make the appointment. Rudy, the scheduler, answered the telephone after seven rings with "Please hold." After what seemed like 20 minutes, he came back on the line and asked what she wanted. Ann replied that she was supposed to have a follow-up visit but no one had yet called to schedule the appointment. Rudy told Ann how busy he was and offered an appointment in three weeks. He reminded her to be early, so they wouldn't have to reschedule if she was late.

On the scheduled date, Ms. Ackney arrives 10 minutes early as instructed for her 8:30 a.m. appointment. Rudy, also the reception-ist, slides back the window and greets her with a curt, "What is your name?"

"Ann Ackney."

"Dr. Frazzle isn't here yet; have a seat," says Rudy as he closes the window and turns to continue socializing with his co-workers. Dr. Frazzle usually sees his first patient at 9 a.m. Today he is doing rounds at the hospital, unaware that Rudy has scheduled an 8:30 appointment.

Ms. Ackney waits until 9:15 and then decides to ask how much longer she must wait. Rudy glares at her and says, "How should I know when he will return to the office? He's always late." Ms. Ackney returns to her chair and decides she will wait 15 minutes more.

At 9:30, Dr. Frazzle walks through the door and greets Ms. Ackney. He walks her back to the exam room, apologizing the entire way. After instructing her to change into a gown, he leaves the exam room and enters his office. His In box is full of telephone messages, several of which he decides to return before seeing Ms. Ackney.

Dr. Frazzle hangs up the telephone. It is now 10 a.m. Again, the first thing he does when he enters the exam room is apologize for being late, explaining that he was on the telephone with a very sick patient. Ms. Ackney wonders why she's not as important as that patient.

He does not have Ms. Ackney's chart, so he apologizes again and asks Ann to review her history for him. She says that she has not heard the test results from her last visit.

Dr. Frazzle leaves the room to ask Bertha, his back-office support staff person, to track down the results of the tests. She learns that the only copy of the results is in Ann's misplaced medical record, so Bertha calls the lab. When she finally gets Ann's results, she has to interrupt Dr. Frazzle to give him the report.

Dr. Frazzle decides he needs to do a procedure, so he reaches into the cupboard for some supplies; which are out of stock. As his frustration level increases, he excuses himself from Ms. Ackney and retrieves the needed supplies from another exam room.

He returns with the supplies, completes the procedure and reviews the diagnosis and treatment plan with Ms. Ackney. Dr. Frazzle leaves the room while she is dressing. He stands behind Bertha and waits for her to get off the telephone. Bertha sees Dr. Frazzle, puts the caller on hold and listens to Dr. Frazzle shout out his orders for Ms. Ackney. He then enters his second patient's exam room – 90 minutes late.

Ms. Ackney leaves the exam room and waits for Bertha to end her telephone conversation. The two discuss Dr. Frazzle's orders before Ann leaves. When she gets to the elevator, she remembers that Dr. Frazzle said he was going to start her on a new medication – however, he did not give her the prescription. She returns to the office and tells Rudy what has happened. Rudy asks her to sit down as he talks to Bertha. Dr. Frazzle is with another patient, so Bertha interrupts Dr. Frazzle again to get the prescription order, which she takes out to Ms. Ackney.

Ann proceeds next to the lab to have her blood drawn. Though Dr. Frazzle said he would call her the next day with the results, she is anxious and worries that he may again forget to call her with the test results. Ann is losing confidence in Dr. Frazzle, not because of his lack of expertise, but because of his chaotic practice. It is disorganized, disconnected and disrespectful.

Finally, when Ann arrives at the pharmacy, the pharmacist tells her he cannot interpret the prescription and must call Dr. Frazzle's office. Ann waits again.

Back at the office, Bertha again interrupts Dr. Frazzle to take the telephone call from the pharmacy. His frustration level is sky high. He shouts the order to the pharmacist with a few unkind words.

Once Ann is home, she forgets Dr. Frazzle's diet instructions. He told her to call back if she had any questions – so she does. Rudy answers the telephone and puts Ms. Ackney on hold before she has a chance to speak. After several minutes, Rudy answers the call again, takes the message and hangs up. Ann waits two hours and hears nothing from the doctor, so she calls again. This time Rudy seems irritated that she is calling a second time. Rudy tells her that Dr. Frazzle is busy and will call her back when he has time. Offended by his tone, Ann hangs up, feeling angry and losing confidence in Dr. Frazzle.

Ms. Ackney's impression of Dr. Frazzle's office:
- They made me wait too long, they don't respect my time;
- They have a rude receptionist;
- They don't really care about me;
- They lost my medical record and test results; I can't trust them to give me good medical care; and
- The doctor seems rushed and frustrated. Is it my fault?

At 7 p.m., Dr. Frazzle finishes with his last patient. He walks into his office and sees a pile of charts that he needs to dictate and the In box again full of telephone messages and mail. He saw 14 patients today – but it seemed like 25. An exhausted Dr. Frazzle feels he is losing control of his practice. He shoves the charge tickets in the charts and leaves for the day, hoping to catch up on his next day off.

Because no one asked about the patients he visited that morning in the hospital, he forgets to charge for those visits.

"Is it worth all this stress?" he wonders.

Work smarter, not harder

As you can see from this story, hard work and devotion alone do not equal a well-run practice.

Not all days go like this day with Dr. Frazzle, but too often care is compromised because of increased frustration in the work place. Lack of information, organization and teamwork leaves patients questioning the competence of their physicians. In addition, when rushed, charges are missed because there is no easy, foolproof system designed to capture charges for procedures performed outside the clinic (and even sometimes inside the clinic).

How do you move from a chaotic practice to an efficient one, or prevent starting your practice on the wrong foot? Chapter 3 provides 7 Guiding Principles for turning chaos into an organized and efficient medical practice. Practice managers must develop systems that support the physician/patient interaction. It is imperative that the entire team, as well as leadership, focus on quality care as perceived by the patient. As you read on, you'll find that you must listen to your patients and focus on efficient systems, real-time work and technology that enhances the practice and adds value for the patient.

CHAPTER 3 | # The 7 Guiding Principles

What we learned from Dr. Frazzle

Dr. Frazzle has a "reactive" practice. When a problem or situation occurs, both the support staff and Dr. Frazzle fly into hyperactive mode and react to the situation, using increased energy and resources. Reactive practices are costly, create little job satisfaction and greatly increase patient dissatisfaction.

A "proactive" practice, on the other hand, does the opposite. It:

- Is controlled and has few surprises;
- Creates job satisfaction;
- Decreases stress levels in the work place;
- Increases patient satisfaction and comfort levels; and
- Promotes teamwork.

Physicians cannot create a proactive environment alone. It takes leadership that understands the operational needs of both the physician and the patient to guide system development and technological implementation to support proactive patient care.

Dr. Frazzle's practice lacks leadership, teamwork, clarity and planning. He does not have a clear vision for his practice; and his support staff does not take responsibility for their jobs or feel part of a greater purpose. If Dr. Frazzle could take the time to analyze his practice and articulate his vision for the practice, his support staff would be empowered to embrace it.

7 Guiding Principles for practice management

Developing systems based on the 7 Guiding Principles could help Dr. Frazzle. He could increase his daily patient volume while gaining control of his practice, and increase patient satisfaction and staff and personal fulfillment. Let these principles guide and enhance your practice. Use them like road maps to keep everyone moving in the appropriate direction and take you on the most efficient and effective route to attaining *your* vision:

- ■■ Work in "real time";
- ■■ Make a time commitment;
- ■■ Balance workloads;
- ■■ Decrease unnecessary variation;
- ■■ Distribute tasks appropriately;
- ■■ Create an interdependent team; and
- ■■ Allocate resources by volume of work.

The proactive approach focuses on planning – anticipating and planning for what may happen.

PRINCIPLE I: Real-time work

Completing work as it presents – or real-time work, including working online – is the most efficient way to operate. Thomas Jefferson said, "Never put off till tomorrow what you can do today." This statement is still true today. Putting work aside to do later increases your error rate and work time, and is one of the major reasons for overtime and/or backlog problems in most practices.

Starting the next workday already behind because of work left over from the previous day adds to the chaos. If you do not have time to do it now, how will you find time to do it later?

Examples of tasks left for another day, also known as "offline work," include:

- Rescheduled patients;
- Messages;
- Dictation;
- Charge capture; and
- Billing.

The visit is a single process that comprises many parts or tasks that are often completed out of sequence. However, learning to complete all work each day enhances practice efficiency and motivates your employees to come back to work every day.

PRINCIPLE II: **Making a time commitment**

Everyone on the health care team must commit to providing timely, value-oriented care. This commitment relates to the amount of time and effort dedicated to seeing patients. It also relates to the time a patient must spend in the office during the entire encounter. Patients value communication with their physicians. They do not value wait time. All tasks must add value to the encounter. Decrease patient wait times, but not the valuable physician face-to-face time with patients.

PRINCIPLE III: **Balancing workloads**

Lack of balance is very costly to a practice; a balanced patient schedule improves service levels, reduces stress and increases patient satisfaction. The easiest way to balance the workload is to schedule the same number of patients each day. Physicians usually see approximately the same number of patients each day; staffing the same number of physicians in the clinic each day will help to balance the volume of work for your staff.

PRINCIPLE IV: Decreasing unnecessary variation

Every practice has necessary and unnecessary variation. Physician practice style is a necessary variation – we do not expect physicians to practice like robots. Style is important and something we do not want to change. Variation of supplies and forms, however, is unnecessary. Standardizing supplies and forms decreases costs. Physicians can usually agree on a standard set of supplies, and where they will be located in each exam room, and rarely is there a good reason to have different vendors for the same supply product. It is important to identify what variation is necessary and what is costly to your practice. Standardization improves patient compliance and consistency of care, and leads to enhanced patient and staff confidence in your practice's system.

PRINCIPLE V: Distributing tasks

Distributing tasks appropriately requires delegating responsibility to the lowest-skill-level person who can perform the task safely and legally. This frees up the physician to spend more time with patients, increases staff job satisfaction and decreases costs. For example, returning phone messages may take the physician an hour or more at the end of the day. Allowing a triage nurse to respond to the call when it comes in gives the physician an extra hour to see patients, and increases physician, patient and nurse satisfaction.

PRINCIPLE VI: Creating an interdependent team

Many management texts document the advantages of teamwork in the work place. People working in teams seem to perform more effectively than people who work alone. Develop forums for staff and physicians to have regular communication – this encourages teamwork.

PRINCIPLE VII: Allocating resources

Allocate resources by volume of work to avoid over- or underutilized staff work time. Staffing levels and number of exam rooms available are the two resources that most affect the efficiency of a patient visit. A high-volume practice needs both more space and support staff than a practice with lower volumes. If a physician sees 30 patients per day, the room turnover time will increase and you will need more staff to keep up with the physician (vs. a physician who sees 15 patients per day). Also, each patient generates a given amount of work; high-volume practices naturally generate more work.

Typical resource allocation per physician is one office, two exam rooms and one support staff person per physician, though this is not always appropriate. In a high-volume practice staff that can't keep up with the physician become the barrier to an efficient practice. Physicians should not wait for staff – the physician limits should be the only barrier.

Chapters 6 though 12 provide detailed information about these principles and ways to implement them in your practice, but before we focus on the details of the principles, we must discuss the importance of mission statements and patient expectations. Remember that patients are your customers and by listening to their needs you will be able to build a successful practice. The mission statement is a tool that helps your patients and staff understand your vision so everyone can work together to assure a viable practice.

CHAPTER 4 | # Best Value in Town

Create a mission statement

In many practice management programs today, physicians chose a mission statement based on being "the best value in town." It is important to focus on value as your patients perceive it, and this entails excellent customer service, appropriate care, quality outcomes, reasonable cost, technology and timely service.

It is also important to identify limitations that prevent having a balanced life. Behaviors that do not support the mission statement are not appropriate – it is not helpful to your patients if you feel frazzled because your practice goals are unattainable. Dr. Frazzle did not have a clearly defined mission statement. If you asked each person on his staff to explain the practice's philosophy or mission, you would get many different answers.

You must analyze where you are going and how you will get there to build a successful practice; this requires input and cooperation from many people, including, first and foremost, your patients. Too often physicians build practices based on their own (sometimes mistaken) perceptions of patients' needs – it is the patients' perceptions that are most important, and the only way you will know your patients' needs is to ask them.

Before you develop your mission statement, you need to ask your patients:

- ■■ What do you want from your physician and the practice?
- ■■ What strengths do you see in our practice?
- ■■ Are we meeting your needs?
- ■■ How can we improve our service to you?

Developing your mission statement

A mission statement explains your reason for existing as a practice in clear, concise, simple terms. A well-written, thoughtfully crafted mission statement can be the basis for evaluating all aspects of your business.

The process of arriving at a mission statement is sometimes as important as the final product, because it causes you to think completely through all aspects of your practice. As part of the process, answer the following questions:

1. Whom do we intend to serve?
2. Why should prospective patients select us over another practice?
3. What do we value?
4. How do we conduct our business?
5. What will we do better than other practices?

As you develop a mission statement, invite the entire staff to participate. The process of asking these questions – especially as a group – can lead to good discussions about your practice's goals, approach to patient care and position in the marketplace. Make sure all physicians in the group, as well as management and staff, agree on the mission. Solicit new ideas. Foster a sense of involvement. To initiate the discussion, you might say, "We want to articulate who we are and what we hope to accomplish in one or two sentences. What are your thoughts?"

A good mission statement often includes the following:

■■ Whom you plan to serve;

■■ What geographic area you will cover;

■■ Your commitment to service;

■■ Your commitment to value; and

■■ How you will resolve disputes.

One clinic printed its mission statement on every appointment card. It began, "Our pledge to you, our patients..." The pledge explained what patients could routinely expect from the practice. It included the clinic's commitment to patient confidentiality, fair pricing, full disclosure and same-day appointments.

Mission statements can be exasperatingly difficult to write; like trying to cram an elephant into a test tube, there seems to be too much to say in a few short sentences. If that happens, focus on thinking about the goals of the practice instead of on wordsmithing. When you clearly think through your goals, the words themselves will come easily enough.

Here is an example:

"Our mission is to provide timely, appropriate and cost-effective health care to patients who require our specialty services and to provide treatment that leads to the best outcomes in a friendly, professional, and patient-focused setting."

One large clinic posted the mission statement in the lobby after every employee signed it. It made a dramatic point of entry and gave a powerful commitment message to each patient who entered.

Too often, mission statements emerge as cold, clinical, passionless platitudes. A mission statement should have heart, soul, zest, and vitality – even humor. It should mirror the personality of the office.

Here are a few more ideas about mission statements:

- ■■ Date them and revisit them annually. Ask your group, "Are we really achieving this mission?" If the answer is yes, celebrate. If you are not achieving your stated mission, either revise your mission statement or change your practice to match the objective.

- ■■ Post your mission statement. Put it where your patients can see it. This helps make you accountable to the people for whom you work – your patients. Seeing it on the wall also is an ever-present reminder to you and your staff of your value system.

- ■■ Make it part of new-staff orientation. Show them the mission statement. Explain how you wrote it. Talk about why you included various aspects in the mission statement.

- ■■ Tie key activities to the mission statement. Use it as a road map for planning and a source of evaluating projects.

When your mission statement is finished, review your patients' expectations, needs and desires, and make sure your mission statement allows you to meet their needs. Remember to define value according to your patients' perceptions.

CHAPTER 5 | # Seeing Your Practice through Your Patients' Eyes

NOW THAT YOU HAVE A MISSION STATEMENT, it is time to determine how you will meet those promises to your patients. Because one tenet of the statement is to meet or exceed patient expectations, you need to determine what your patients expect from your practice.

Identify patient expectations

Let us put first things first. Patients are the reason your medical practice exists. Ultimately, patients help you succeed or fail. Successful practices build their systems based on patients' desires and needs.

We recommend three approaches to identifying patients' expectations:

1. Write a patient satisfaction survey.
2. Conduct patient focus groups to obtain direct input about patient expectations. Focus groups take more time, but there is no substitute for talking directly with patients.

3. Use e-mail. Your patients arrive home from your office to find an e-mail asking them to provide feedback on their experience and expressing your appreciation for the opportunity to care for them. Using protected e-mail gives you real-time open communication with your patients – the perfect opportunity for continual quality improvement.

Does this sound simple? It is. But in the hubbub of setting up a practice, hiring staff and developing systems, it is easy to overlook the patients' interests. It is easy, while scurrying from exam room to exam room, to lose sight of the singular impression each patient takes away from his or her visit.

The practice team that understands and meets or exceeds patient desires will have a growing, satisfied patient base, and in fact, most patients' expectations are modest. A positive attitude sometimes can compensate for disorganization. A warm smile and helpful approach will ease most situations. Here is a patient wish list compiled from our patient satisfaction surveys and focus groups. Meeting each of these requests is easy to achieve.

I am your patient, I want you to:
- Know my name;
- See me promptly;
- Make me comfortable;
- Tell me what's happening;
- Have everything ready for my visit; and
- Bill me quickly and correctly.

The importance of names

The most beautiful word in a person's language is his or her own name. Calling a person by name immediately shows recognition, respect and concern. Encourage every member of the team to use patient names. Always use the formal approach, Mr. Smith or Ms. Martin, unless the patient gives you permission to use his or her first name.

Similarly, patients like to know with whom they are dealing. All staff members need to wear a badge that includes his or her first name and title. Patients often believe they are speaking to a registered nurse when, in fact, they are talking to a clerical support person or with a physician when they are talking with a physician's assistant. Remember also to use your name and title when using other kinds of communication, like e-mail. It is unfair to let patients assume they are hearing from the physician when in actuality it is the medical assistant. Do not be afraid to say, "Dr. Efficient requested that I e-mail you and let you know..." Patients do not mind hearing from support staff as long as they realize which person directed the correspondence.

Appropriate and timely scheduling

If you want to surprise and delight your patients when they call the office, offer them a same-day appointment. This type of scheduling is becoming the norm today. When you see patients on the day they call, the visit is usually shorter and more focused, and patient satisfaction is higher.

Access to the Internet has opened up a new venue for patients to schedule their own appointments. No longer do they have to wait on hold or use clinic resources to schedule an appointment. Let them do it themselves. This sounds scary; but it can work smoothly – and consider the money you will save in staff time.

Imagine if a mother wakes at 7 a.m. to find her child has a fever. Instead of calling the answering service (who forwards the call to the physician who then calls the patient to tell her to call the office at 8 a.m.), she goes to her computer, pulls up your practice's website and schedules an appointment that is both convenient for her and meets your scheduling rules. As she clicks on the reason for the visit, another window appears that gives her treatments she might want to try at home before bringing her child into the office. The Internet also offers an opportunity for patient education. Well-informed patients are more compliant and take up less resource time.

Appealing waiting area

Patients expect clean and neat waiting areas; they appreciate comfortable chairs that they can get in and out of easily. We often hear patients complain about outdated reading material, poor lighting and too much clutter in waiting rooms. Most patients do not like offices that are too fancy, because they wonder if the physician's fees could be lower if it weren't for the nicely decorated office. Remember to display copies of your practice brochure, patient education materials and physician and nurse biographies for your patients to read and know that you care about them and want to keep them informed.

Communicating about delays

Most patients will wait patiently for about 15 minutes. If the wait is longer than that, tell the patient why there is a delay. When you are honest, patients will usually understand especially if the office is handling an emergency or a difficult case. However, if delays or long waits occur consistently, they will lose confidence in your practice – and may even begin to show up late to counteract their wait time.

With new technology, you can hand your patients an electronic tablet and have them complete their "paperwork" online as they wait. Your patients could input all their demographic and health history information into your system while they are waiting. This saves resource time, decreases misinterpretation of information and assures you of having current information as soon as the non-physician provider or physician walks in the exam room – and as a bonus, the patients' wait passed quickly for them.

Alternatively, patients can fill out a bubble form and your office can scan it into your system – either way you have instant accurate information – however, having patients fill out paper forms creates added work for your staff, increases chance of errors by misinterpreting handwriting, precludes you having the information at the time of the visit, so you must ask all the information again, and the billing is often delayed.

Exam room protocol for physicians

> **KEY:** Enter the exam room prepared.

LISTEN TO THE PATIENTS. Give them time to tell their story. It will take them only two minutes or so to tell you all of their concerns. Knowing all the issues up front will allow you to better judge the time available for each issue. This way you can take control and address all the issues in the order of importance to you. This will eliminate that "one last question" as you are walking out the door.

SHOW CONCERN. Your patients will perceive you as caring with three simple behaviors: have eye contact, listen attentively, and call them by name.

PRESENT OPTIONS. Patients value honest and full disclosure. Give the facts and present various options. Allow the patient to be a partner in making treatment decisions, or at least explain why you are taking a certain course and what options you eliminated and why.

PUT IT IN WRITING. During exams, many patients are a bundle of nerves. They may forget almost everything you have said, so write down all treatment plans. (Imagine pushing one button to print a visit summary for the patient that includes pertinent patient education material.) Encourage the patient to keep copies of their records and to monitor their health status periodically.

BRING CLOSURE. Let the patient – not you – end the exam. Before you leave, answer questions, listen and ask, "Have you received what you needed today?"

EHR benefits

The electronic health record (EHR) provides a one-page form that comprises a few lines of personal information about the patient and a list of all their visits, tests and medications – basically a one-page summary that covers years of care. It is possible with the EHR to eliminate the embarrassing fumble through the paper chart looking for facts, trying to piece together a patient's history and trying to remember the patient. Never again will you have to see a patient without the complete chart.

Many patients say they find it disconcerting when their physician asks questions that indicate the physician is not aware of their case. The EHR, which can display all the important information on a one-page summary sheet that includes a list of the patient's health problems, treatments, medications, and family, social and medical histories, saves physicians valuable time and enables them to recall the patient quickly – restoring patient confidence. Physicians can share the electronic chart with the patient to relieve any anxiety.

Timely follow-up

When physicians order tests, patients want to hear the results as soon as possible. If the patient is ill, has had a procedure, or is anxious, a courtesy call to see how the patient is doing will build confidence in the physician and the system.

Communicate test results. Send normal test results in writing by the time promised. If the results are abnormal, call the patient immediately. Explain the results and any required follow-up appointments or procedures. Patients worry. They will call many times if you do not take control of the process and arrange for a time to get results back to them. Leaving a message to call the office often scares patients. Do not leave messages late in the day or on Friday afternoons, unless you can be available to answer calls after business hours. Patients always imagine the worst if they cannot reach the physician or nurse. Be aware of confidentiality issues when leaving a message on an answering device or on a voicemail. (Also, make sure the patient gave permission to leave a message and document this permission in the record.) Being able to access test results any time on the Internet would eliminate the patient's anxious wait for the results. It also will decrease the time your staff spends copying and mailing results or calling patients with the results.

Now imagine if, from the comfort of your home office, while waiting for the kids to wake up for a family breakfast, Dr. Efficient goes to the computer and sees a list of all test results from yesterday. A click on each test shows if it is normal, another click files the results in the chart and sends a copy to the patient via e-mail. Action buttons are there for test results requiring more activity. Dr. Efficient can send a prescription to the patient's pharmacy and an e-mail to the patient, or call the patient and schedule an appointment – and then join his or her family for breakfast.

Make courtesy telephone calls or e-mails. Identify key patients each day to call or e-mail the following day. Usually one or two patients will stand out each day as significant because they had a procedure or because they were extremely anxious. The criterion each physician uses to identify key patients is not as important as remembering to call or e-mail them each day to see how they are doing. Patients truly appreciate personal communication.

Appropriate and timely billing

Patients expect clear communication about the bill due date, acceptable forms of payment, who can answer questions or discuss concerns and what number to call if they have questions.

Send out statements that are clear and easy to understand. Your patients should not need a Masters in Business Administration to figure how much they owe or a Masters in Public Health to understand the services they received.

We often hear staff say, "Patients should know what amount their insurance pays, that's not our responsibility." Although that's probably true, it is good customer service and in the best interest of the practice to help the patient understand their responsibility and then ask for payment before the patient leaves the office. Collect all you can up front. The more you can do up front, the less rework your staff will have later in the billing office.

The electronic medium has revolutionized the billing process. We now have the tools to identify patient portions, and we can help patients identify in real time what the out-of-pocket responsibilities will be before they leave the office. (Dentists have done this for years.)

Imagine that within moments after a patient makes an appointment, your office automatically receives confirmation about the patient's insurance and the portion the patient needs to pay. Once you document the visit, the system automatically bills the insurance company. Reimbursement arrives within days – just another benefit of the EHR.

The following chapters will guide you through a process of developing essential systems that a successful medical practice needs. It is important that management, physicians and staff work together to develop practical systems that support efficient, effective patient care. It also is important that patients perceive value from each interaction with your organization.

Read on with an open mind. Think about how you can use the 7 Guiding Principles to improve the value of care your patients receive and maintain a more balanced and enjoyable practice for you and your staff. Do not be afraid to dream of what it could be like in a perfect world.

CHAPTER 6

PRINCIPLE I

Real-time Work

REAL-TIME WORK MEANS DOING TODAY'S WORK TODAY. Don't procrastinate. It's a difficult feat, but one that will bring endless satisfaction, let alone monetary rewards, back into your practice.

It is usually efficient to receive care at an urgent care center; indeed, many patients use urgent care clinics as their primary care providers because the clinic operates efficiently. Urgent care clinics use – for the most part – real-time work. They see patients as they come in, complete the entire visit at the time the patient is there and collect for the visit as the patient leaves.

We realize that each practice is different, but it is startling to consider how the typical practice can generate so much work trying to control its internal processes. The additional work adds cost and is unlikely to keep your practice in control. Most clinics function as separate departments, a front office, back office and billing department. Each sets its own rules and tries to control the process in its own area, often times inadvertently sabotaging the other areas. As problems arise, new policies are added until chaos rules.

A patient encounter is a single system from the phone call until payment is received. Unfortunately, we have taken a straightforward process and turned it into a complex, inefficient string of processes. This must change and the first step is to simplify your processes. Look at your practice as a single system. Build processes that allow for real-time work. Technology allows us to do more real-time work (as long as we can trust the system).

The following are examples of real-time work:
- ■ Allow patients to schedule their own appointments;
- ■ Let patients input their demographics and health history;
- ■ Verify insurance at the time of appointment;
- ■ Have someone qualified to answer medical and insurance questions answer phone calls;
- ■ Collect co-pays and patient portions up front;
- ■ Complete visit documentation at the time of the visit;
- ■ Schedule follow-up visits, order and authorize tests and give patient treatment plan and educational information before leaving the exam room;
- ■ Code and bill charges at time of visit;
- ■ Bill today's charges today; and
- ■ Do today's work today.

If there is one change that will most influence your practice, it is adopting the real-time work concept. Technology makes it easier to accomplish more work in a real-time manner. A good EHR will force you to do real-time work. At day's end, you will feel rewarded and relieved you don't have to start the next workday behind.

Working in real time is the first step in making a time commitment to your patients. It's a promise to use their time and your time efficiently and effectively.

The other Guiding Principles take real-time work into account and Chapter 14 provides an example of real-time work in action. You will see the immediate rewards one practice reaps after it implements this Guiding Principle.

CHAPTER 7

PRINCIPLE II
Making a Time Commitment

REAL-TIME WORK ALLOWS YOU TO BEGIN TO ANALYZE how you use your time. In the past schedules had little to do with the daily work volume, since much of the work done today was from yesterday, last week or even last month. By working in real time, you gain control of your practice and can begin to plan and use your time more effectively. Once you can plan your time efficiently, you can make a time commitment to your patients, yourself and your staff – a promise to respect their time and use it wisely.

Making a time commitment relates to two different measurements of time. One is the time the physician commits to his/her practice, and the other is the time it takes a patient to flow through your system – from check-in to check-out. It is all about managing time – your time and your patient's time. For our explanation, we will use a clinic-based practice, but this Guiding Principle is true for any practice. Determining the amount of time each physician will spend in the clinic seeing patients is the first step in making a time commitment to the practice. Making this commitment is the conscious and deliberate act of deciding how many hours each physician plans to be available to see patients day-by-day, week-by-week and year-by-year.

Time, after all, is the "product" that physicians sell in their practice. The amount of time physicians choose to spend at the practice is up to each physician. However, it is vitally important to make a commitment in specific, measurable terms. Productivity relates directly to each physician's time commitment. Committing a set number of hours to each physician's practice does not guarantee that patients will fill each open slot. It does however give you a measurable target, a place to start and an important benchmark for practice measurement.

Taking a time inventory will also help you calculate the resource level needed to support each physician. Work volume directly relates to the time each physician allocates for seeing patients. Low productivity often relates to excess time away from the office.

Over the last 20 years, we have noticed that several physicians with dwindling practices simply spent too much time out of the office. If you carefully document each physician's time away from the office, you will know exactly the number of days per year each physician should spend in the clinic, seeing patients.

Physician time in the clinic

How do you calculate the time each physician will spend in the office? Simply start with the number of days in a year, then reduce that number by subtracting weekends, vacation days, holidays and professional development seminars days.

It is amazing how fast 365 days dwindle. An example is shown in Figure 7.1.

According to these calculations, each physician should work 215 days per year in the clinic, seeing patients. You can begin to determine from this information how many patients per day each physician must see to meet his or her goal.

Start with an annual calendar and determine each physician's basic schedule. It sounds impossible, but it's not.

FIGURE 7.1 **Available Clinic Days Worksheet**

AVAILABLE CLINIC DAYS
(Sample Worksheet)

365	Total days per year
−104	Weekend days
−6	Holidays
−20	Vacation days
−20	Professional days
215	Available clinic days

Begin by setting the schedule rules for each practice. These are rules that dictate the number of physicians and other providers that work in the practice each day.

- ▪▪ Who: Which physicians and providers see which types of patients?
- ▪▪ What: Which type(s) of patients does your practice see?
- ▪▪ When: What are clinic hours? Hospital hours? Call hours?
- ▪▪ Where: Is the patient seen in the hospital or at the clinic?
- ▪▪ How: The rules of 'how to care' for patients are set by the Who, What, When and Where of your practice.

Here are some simple tools to help you build an annual, balanced schedule.

1. Put up a dry-erase 12-month calendar on the wall and have physicians mark out the days they plan to be out of the office over the next year, including who gets which holidays off, meetings, vacations, etc.

2. Then prepare a call schedule.

3. Determine the minimum number of providers in the office each day.

4. Last, set up a work schedule.

Realize that there may be some changes, but this process begins to have physicians work their personal lives around their practice obligations. This process allows you to plan the year. Knowing the number of days each provider will be in the clinic is the first step.

Patient-visit revenue

Determine the revenue generated from each patient visit. Remember this is revenue generated, not actual revenue. For example, in a surgery practice, a certain number of visits equals one surgery. Include all the surgery revenue.

Use the sample information in Figure 7.2 to calculate the revenue generated per visit.

If a physician wants higher annual compensation, for example, $280,000, divide that figure by the predetermined per-visit

FIGURE 7.2 **Sample Calculations for Revenue Generated per Visit**

Annual gross charges per physician	$1,000,000
Annual collections per physician	$500,000
Annual overhead 50%	$250,000
Annual compensation per physician	$250,000
Annual visits	4,000
Average physician compensation per visit	$62.50

compensation figure (280,000/62.50) and you see that the doctor needs to generate 4,480 visits annually. Don't forget to include a percentage for "no-shows." Is this possible in your practice?

Let us assume for easy math that the goal is 4,500 office visits per year per physician and that each physician plans to see those patients in 215 days. That equals 21 patients per day per physician. If each physician averages two no-shows per day and if you add those two to the 21 patients actually seen each day, each physician's goal per day would be 23 scheduled patient-care visits.

The sample worksheet in Figure 7.3 demonstrates how to calculate the number of scheduled patient-care visits needed per day.

FIGURE 7.3 **Patient-care Visits per Day Worksheet**

OFFICE VISIT GOALS
(Sample Worksheet)

4,500	Total annual office visits
Divided by 215	Available days
Equals 21	Average patients per day
Plus 2	Average "no-shows" per day
Equals 23	Average scheduled office visits per day
Times 20 minutes per patient	Average minutes per visit
Equals 460 minutes per day	Average minutes
Divided by 60 equals 7.7 hours of time that needs to be scheduled per day	Available hours per day

This example demonstrates the identification process for available hours of scheduled time per day to accomplish the compensation goal within a set number of days. To complete the worksheet, you must first identify the average length of time a physician spends with each patient.

Continuous stopwatch time study

You can use several different methods to determine the average length of time physicians spend per patient. In our studies, we use the Continuous Stopwatch Time Study methodology, which uses an outside observer who actually watches and records the time each physician spends with each patient. This method is more accurate than self-analysis tools or using average times from the schedule. The time study also gives you the opportunity to identify all the components of a patient visit, not just the face-to-face time. For our studies, we include the following tasks in a patient visit:

- ■■ Reviewing the chart;
- ■■ Spending face-to-face time with the patient;
- ■■ Dictating the patient visit into the record;
- ■■ Completing the chart and charge ticket;
- ■■ Talking with family members; and
- ■■ Reviewing test results with patients and staff.

A continuous study means you start the stopwatch as the physician begins in the morning and stop it once he or she finishes in the evening. Each time the physician changes tasks, you record the task. Record the time used to complete each task.

When the study is complete, calculate the time per task by subtracting the beginning task time from the ending task time. Review all task times on a summary sheet and record the total number of patients seen. If you divide the number of patients into the six tasks in a complete patient visit, you will arrive at the average number of minutes per patient visit.

Figure 7.4 illustrates how task time is calculated.

FIGURE 7.4 **Calculation for Time Required per Task**

TASK	TIME	TOTAL TASK TIME
Start time	8:00 a.m.	
Task 1 Check in	Completed 8:05 a.m.	5 minutes
Task 2 Room patient	Completed 8:10 a.m.	5 minutes
Task 3 Doctor in exam room	Completed 8:30 a.m.	20 minutes
Task 4 Patient check out	Completed 8:40 a.m.	10 minutes
Total patient time		40 minutes

Figure 7.5 demonstrates how to calculate average patient visit time.

FIGURE 7.5 **Calculation of Average Time per Patient Visit**

TASK	TOTAL TIME	AVERAGE TIME PER TASK
Check-in	100 minutes	5 minutes
Room patient	110 minutes	5.5 minutes
Physician with patient	450 minutes	22.5 minutes
Checkout	120 minutes	6 minutes
Conclusion	20 patients seen	Average time per patient visit is 39 minutes

Self-analysis tool

A second method for acquiring time information is a self-analysis tool, shown in Figure 7.6. While this method is not as accurate as the stopwatch method, physicians can complete the task

independently. Attach the following form to each chart and monitor physician time for several weeks. Begin recording task times
when the patient goes into the exam room. Note the time each person interacts with the patient and record the time under the "in"
column. Also, record the time each person leaves the room under
the "out" column. Subtract the "out" column from the "in" column
to arrive at your task time. Do this procedure for all tasks.

FIGURE 7.6 **Task Time Self-Analysis Tool**

SELF-ANALYSIS TOOL

TASK	TIME IN	TIME OUT	TASK TIME
Patient			
Nurse			
Physician			
Dictation/charting/ charge ticket			
Review test results			

If the average time each physician spends with each patient visit is
20 minutes, each physician will need 460 minutes or 7.7 hours of
available patient-care time per day, as shown in the original worksheet. This is feasible.

Remember to monitor the number of days physicians actually work
in the clinic seeing patients and the number of patients seen each
day. The major reason for decreased annual revenue is working
fewer days than the calculated number of days per year and/or seeing fewer patients per day than the goal.

As basic as this groundwork sounds, many physicians do not know how many days they worked in the clinic last year, let alone how many patients they saw. When physicians guess at the number of patients they see per week, the number is invariably high. Physicians tend to think back to their busiest days, and then project that same volume to the rest of the schedule.

In declining practices, failure to monitor patient volumes and days worked are common problems. If, for example, you averaged 20 patients per day in 2000, 19 in 2001, 18 in 2002, 17 in 2003, etc., you would probably not feel the decrease over a five-year period. However, your practice would decrease by 25 percent, a rather substantial loss, and you probably would not realize this fact until it was too late.

Have a plan for the year. Set a patient goal per day to benefit the physician by providing the perfect yardstick for measuring productivity.

A time inventory allows you to:
- ∎∎ Plan staff annual needs;
- ∎∎ Forecast annual revenue by estimating dollars-per-visit times number of visits;
- ∎∎ Share tangible productivity goals with staff;
- ∎∎ Motivate staff to maintain a full schedule;
- ∎∎ Allocate staff-to-patient volume; and
- ∎∎ Balance the workload.

It is imperative not only to identify the number of hours each physician will spend in the clinic each week, but also to monitor his or her accessibility. If patients call and are told the next appointment is weeks away, something is wrong.

Support-staff barriers

Each week support staff should identify how long it is until the physician's third next-available appointment. We often see practices that have time to see patients; but schedule barriers make it difficult to set timely patient appointments. Sometimes the amount of work the support staff can handle limits the physicians' ability to see more patients. Too few support staff may be the problem, but more often it is the result of having an unbalanced practice. This is not acceptable. Never limit a practice by the amount of work your support staff can handle.

Another common limitation we see is support staff protecting a physician by limiting the number of patients seen in one day. Staff members often protect the schedule out of concern for the physician or themselves. Unfortunately, we have seen times when the support staff has literally "protected" the physician out of business.

Closing your practice to new patients

It is very dangerous, especially in today's environment, to close a practice to new patients. Practices limit themselves. When appointment access reaches a level that is not acceptable to patients, they will seek care elsewhere. Patients leave for various reasons; oftentimes the physician and staff are never aware of the change. Physicians who close their practices to new patients for as little as six months often have a difficult time rebuilding the practice.

Patient throughput vs. perceived value

Another time-commitment measure is patient throughput, or the time it takes a patient to complete each task between check-in and checkout, including all wait times. Tracking this information will let you know how efficient your practice is and where the bottlenecks are located. Patients consider time with someone productive and wait times non-productive, so the ratio between the two is what we measure.

For example, if a patient checked in at 1:30 p.m. and checked out at 3:45 p.m., we would say their throughput time was 2 hours and 15 minutes. However, if you measured each interval time (see Figure 7.7) and the total time face-to-face with either a physician or staff member was only 20 minutes, we would say their productive time ratio was only 15 percent. The higher this number, the better. The wait time was 85 percent of this visit. Patients prefer no wait time – 0 percent.

Monitor throughput periodically by attaching the form shown in Figure 7.7 to each chart for one week. Synchronize all watches and clocks in the practice.

FIGURE 7.7 **Monitoring Throughput Time**

Appointment time	1:00 p.m.
Check-in time	12:55 p.m.
Chart-up time	1:00 p.m.
Taken-to-room time	1:20 p.m.
Chart-on-door time	1:25 p.m.
Doctor-in time	2:00 p.m.
Doctor-out time	2:10 p.m.
Check-out time	2:15 p.m.

The throughput time on the above patient, when using the appointment time to check-out time ratio, is 75 minutes. By using check-in time to check-out time, as purists would, the throughput time is 80 minutes. However, the face-to-face time is only 20 minutes; therefore, the patient would perceive value for only 25 percent of the visit.

All the methodologies in this chapter measured time. They have proven to be very effective, but time consuming. With the right EHR, you could identify any statistical measurement you chose at any time. For example, you could click on an icon and learn:

■■ How long you spent with each patient;

■■ How many patients you have seen compared to your goal;

■■ How long it takes to room a patient;

■■ How long patients wait in the lobby or the exam room; and

■■ Your no-show rate.

Letting your system continually measure your work and your staff's work will help you make the needed process adjustments in a timely manner with little effort spent collecting data. EHRs have the ability to time-stamp every action and calculate the results on a real-time basis.

Remember that making a time commitment is invaluable, but unless you balance practice workloads, you will not be able to maximize your time and keep that commitment.

CHAPTER 8

PRINCIPLE III
Balancing Workloads

A BALANCED WORKLOAD
IS THE KEY TO A SUCCESSFUL PRACTICE.

Scheduling approximately the same number of physicians available on any given day results in predictable workloads for the practice. This leads to steady, measured support-staff use and helps set the framework for a steady daily patient flow. Balance can make the difference between a smoothly run and a chaotic practice.

Use the annual schedule discussed in the Chapter 7 to balance the number of providers in the clinic at any given time. Staffing the same number of physicians day to day evenly distributes workloads throughout the week. It will never be perfect, but in practices without balanced physician coverage, wild daily capacity fluctuations can occur. If you have four providers and the ideal number in the clinic is three, then aim for having three providers in clinic 80 percent of the time and the other 20 percent have no more than four and no fewer than two. Note that on the days when you have only two physicians onsite, you will need to send staff home or increase the cost per visit. On the days when you have four providers, you will be short staffed, and rooms and wait times will increase – all of which are costly to your practice. It is easy to overlook uneven physician staffing levels when diagnosing a dysfunctional practice – but often it is a contributing factor.

This uncertainty – the feast or famine in patient flow – turns work into a roller coaster for the staff. It's no wonder the staff at such practices are edgy, uptight and often curt with patients.

The patient, who ultimately bears the brunt for this planning failure, is rushed through the system, left unattended in the exam room, or ignored for too long in the waiting room. A patient who experiences this rude treatment from clinic staff members may not say anything immediately, but there are studies that show that when a person experiences poor service, he or she will tell 27 other people about it. "The long wait" will be the topic of many dinner conversations, party tidbits, and an agenda item when a friend asks for a physician referral. "I can tell you where *not* to go," will be the answer. This is word-of-mouth advertising gone amok.

Fundamentally, uneven staffing increases the chance of providing inconsistent or poor service to patients, who are the very reason a practice exists.

In smaller practices, balanced staffing occurs informally. "Oh, you are taking your vacation then. Well, I will schedule mine a few weeks after you return."

In medium-sized practices, where communication among providers is not as personal or frequent, problems start to occur; often in large multi-specialty clinics, no single person knows the onsite physician roster on any given day.

The solution: select a central person to manage a clinic-wide master schedule to track staffing every single day of the year. Structure the schedule to guarantee even coverage while accommodating vacations, professional development, research and other activities.

The staffing must be adequate to sustain a balanced patient flow through the practice. Who suffers the most on the days that you are either over- or understaffed? In the short run, the patient suffers, but physicians and staff members also feel the pain. It will not be long until the entire practice suffers. Word will get out that this practice does not provide good service.

Take a moment and see how this works in practice. The graph in Figure 8.1 shows volumes of daily visits in a practice where day-to-day variations range from 84 to 178 patient visits. This particular clinic scheduled the same support staff each day. What should the accurate staffing volume be? The mathematical average is 120 patients per day (shown as the trend line in Figure 8.1). If that actually held true, about one-third of the time the practice would be short-staffed. If one person checks in all your patients and your volume rises from 84 to 176 patient visits, there will be a queue in the waiting area. On the days when the volume drops, there are wasted labor hours.

FIGURE 8.1 **Example of Daily Staffing Variables**

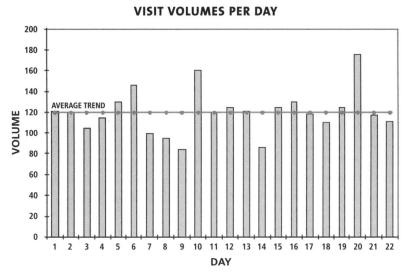

A copy of a balanced master schedule is shown in Figure 8.2. Balanced staffing makes good business sense. It avoids staff turnover and assures astute labor use. It is also good for physicians

FIGURE 8.2 **Example of Balanced Master Schedule**

MASTER SCHEDULE

Dr.	Mon. a.m.	Mon. p.m.	Tue. a.m.	Tue. p.m.	Wed. a.m.	Wed. p.m.	Thu. a.m.	Thu. p.m.	Fri. a.m.	Fri. p.m.
Dr. A	CL	CL	OR	OR	CL	CL	CL	CL	Off	Off
Dr. B	Off	Off	OR	CL	CL	CL	CL	CL	CL	CL
Dr. C	CL	CL	CL	OR	Off	Off	OR	OR	CL	CL
NP			CL	CL				CL		
MW							CL			
CL	2	2	2	2	2	2	3	3	2	2

CL=In clinic; OR = In surgery; NP = Nurse practitioner; MW = Midwife

because they can operate in a more predictable environment without feeling rushed and pushed; however, most important, keeping a balanced master schedule results in good service to your patients.

Many practices use part-time physicians or nonphysician providers to help balance the schedule. A practice where part-time providers choose to work the same days as the full-time providers can suffer imbalance because the part-time workers fail to fill in the valleys and only add to the peak days.

Patient demand affects schedule balance. More patients call on Mondays wanting same-day appointments than any other day of the week yet Monday schedules are usually full. When you squeeze extra patients in on Monday and then they need a follow-up visit, do not schedule their return visit on one of your busiest call-in days.

If you don't address the visit volume balance in your practice, you will continue to have daily volume variations that over time will add unnecessary stress to you and your staff, long patient wait times and unnecessary costs. With a little planning, your productivity will improve as will the atmosphere of your practice.

By following the steps below, balancing your workload will be easy:

- ▪▪ Build a year-out schedule having all providers identify the time they will be away from the practice during the year. There may be some changes along the way each year, but 80 percent correct is better than guessing;

- ▪▪ Establish master schedule rules;

- ▪▪ Set the call schedule;

- ▪▪ Build a standard work schedule for each provider. There will be some standard rotation; if not weekly, it may be every other week or monthly, but there will be a pattern. Find the pattern and repeat it throughout the year;

- ▪▪ Add the number of providers on each half day. Work with the providers to smooth out the peaks and valleys; and

- ▪▪ Set the schedule in stone except for emergencies. Generally, don't allow changes to the schedule within 90 days, except for emergencies.

Another solution by which your practice can automatically balance its workload is by adopting the "open-access concept," whereby patients are seen when they want to be seen and by the provider of choice. This concept will be discussed in the next chapter.

CHAPTER 9

PRINCIPLE IV

Decreasing Unnecessary Variation

VARIATION IS COSTLY. It is important that you lay the groundwork for smooth practice operations by decreasing unnecessary variation within your organization.

When new physicians join a practice, more often than not managers ask the physicians to design their own practice systems. Most physicians tend to develop very different systems or ways to handle the operations of the practice because they have no idea how others handle the same situation, though when asked, they will devise a solution. It is far better to ask physicians what their needs and expectations are for different systems. Show them how your organization completes tasks and let them respond if they need something done differently. Most physicians tell us that they really do not care how work is done as long as the job is completed correctly and in a timely manner; rarely do they want to design systems themselves – they want to see patients.

Long before scheduling the first appointment, implement systems that will make the best use of each physician's time. (Of course, in existing practices, it is never too late to put new systems in place.) Ask your physicians what they need from various systems. Standardizing will improve physician productivity and decrease costs.

Scheduling rules

Scheduling problems usually are the result of inconsistent practice patterns and scheduling rules. Too often, physicians' scheduling rules change based on the mood of the day. This is difficult for the staff, who feel defeated because they never seem to be able to establish a consistent, hard-fast schedule. Having clear, understandable and consistent scheduling rules allows staff to meet physician needs when scheduling appointments. When developing scheduling rules remember fewer rules are better. Here are the steps:

FIGURE 9.1 **Example of Scheduling Rules**

Provider	Day of the Week	Basic Clinic Schedule	Call Day Rules	Non-call Day Rules
Dr. A	Monday Tuesday Wednesday Thursday Friday	Clinic Surgery Off Clinic Call	Only short visits, 3 per hour. Can add one short visit per hour if necessary.	Short visits 10 minutes. Long visits 20 minutes. Fill first hour each day with follow-up patients.
Dr. B	Monday a.m. Monday p.m. Tuesday Wednesday Thursday Friday	Clinic Satellite Clinic Surgery Clinic Call Clinic	Only short visits, 3 per hour. Can add one short visit per hour if necessary.	Short visits 15 minutes. Long visits 30 minutes. Fill first hour each day with follow-up patients.
General Rules		Clinic hours 8 a.m.–noon and 1:30 p.m.–5:30 p.m.		Offer every patient the option of a same day visit.

FIRST, call a brainstorming meeting of all the physicians who will be practicing together and using the same support staff. In a large group practice, the meeting might involve a specialty or a section.

SECOND, group patients by length of appointment time in two basic categories – long and short. Agree on which patients require less time and which need more.

Use this meeting to develop scheduling rules, categorize appointments by length of time it takes for the physician to see the patient, and to identify criteria for the outliers – indicators that cause particular patients to take more time, such as a patient on 10 different medications or one who has seen multiple physicians over the past year. This helps assure the staff will schedule appointments appropriately. Note that the rules can be simple, as shown in Figure 9.1.

Develop three simple questions the receptionists can ask to determine if the patient falls in the extended visit category. Another benefit of the electronic health record is that once a physician sees a patient, the provider can determine that a particular patient always needs more time and then can annotate that recurrent need in the record.

A schedule is simply a tool to help organize your day, not an absolute. Trying to determine the exact time it takes to see each patient is difficult. Many clinics have as few as 10 or as many as 200 different appointment types; but of course this only adds chaos to the practice. Appointment lengths, once more consistent, are now more dependent on the patient than on the reason for the visit – a change from what we saw 10 years ago. We don't know if this happens because of an increase in behavioral health issues that affect many practices (limited resources are usually a factor for physicians seeking treatment) or because patients tend to switch physicians more often than in years past (due to changes in health insurance policies and limited plans). This does mean that it's important to identify those patients who need more time with the physician and practice staff.

THIRD, identify the reasons you see most patients. Put each of these visits into no more than three categories; short, medium or long. Most physicians use two categories (for example, 15 minutes and 30 minutes), though we are seeing more physicians who see all patients using one time frame – their schedules are built around seeing three patients per hour (for instance), regardless of the reason for the visit. This works well for some physicians, and is easy for the schedulers.

The time physicians choose to see patients will be different for each physician and should meet the physician's practice style. Consistency can be imposed with the type of patients seen in each category. For instance, a person coming in for a physical with no problems can be scheduled under the same category for all physicians. The type of visit chart shown in Figure 9.2 shows how you can have the same appointment categories and yet each physician can assign the length of time appropriate for her or his style.

FIGURE 9.2 **Physician Time Spent by Visit Type**

TYPE OF VISIT IN MINUTES

	Brief (BV)	Intermediate (IV)	Extended (EV)	Comprehensive (CV)	Complex (CX)
MD 1	10	20	30	40	50
MD2	10	10	20	20	30

Discuss whether you can provide a particular service in a short, medium or long visit. While some compromise is necessary, natural groupings of visits by the amount of time they require typically emerge. Use only physician time to determine appointment length. (Often we see appointment times built with support time included. This is another example of letting your support-staff time dictate patient volume instead of your desire and availability to see patients.)

FOURTH, decide what is unique about each of these appointment categories. Some practices define new patients as unique, because a new set of data is created and developed for each one. Consultations are usually unique because you not only need to build a new database, but you also must review outside records. Build criteria for patients that fall under each category.

Be sure to standardize the Remarks column as seen in Figure 9.3 below. Abbreviations can mean many things, so choose the ones you want to use in your practice. Place standardized key information

FIGURE 9.3 **Appointment Criteria**

Abbreviation	Appointment name	Description	Remarks
New	New Patient visit	New database evaluation.	Date of last physical.
Con	Consult	Referred from another provider or seeking a second opinion.	Referring provider/ have outside records been ordered/date of last exam/problem.
BV	Brief visit	Simple problem, for instance, rash, conjunctivitis, earache, sore throat, cough, wound check, post op or follow-up to recent visit.	Primary care provider/chief complaint/duration.
EV	Extended visit	Multiple problems, new patients not wanting a complete evaluation, return database evaluation or any problem not listed under BV.	Date of last exam/ list problems or state no problems.

in a field that anyone looking at the schedule can use and understand. This is the information the back office support staff will need
when preparing the chart and room for the patient visit.
Remember, the proactive approach saves physician time.

FIFTH, each physician assigns the length of time he or she needs for
each of these visit categories. The time must match practice style.
For example, a physician who works swiftly may allow 10 minutes
for short appointments, while another provider who likes to spend
more time may allocate 15 minutes for short visits. Don't schedule
physicians for 10 minutes if they need 15 – the result will be long
waits for the patients and frustrated physicians.

Appointment types

If you build appropriate appointment types, you can develop logi-
cal thought processes to help the staff schedule more effectively.
This process is a rules-based approach to appointment scheduling.

Here are the benefits of going through this exercise:

- It helps the telephone staff move logically from a caller's
  need, to reason for visit, to criteria for visit and then to allocate the appropriate amount of time for any type of appointment;
- It allows flexibility for physicians to write rules that help
  direct questions to the patient so that the answers automatically place a patient in a particular appointment type;
- It allows for accurate centralized or decentralized scheduling
  and restores physician confidence in the schedulers; and
- It also gives physicians the trust to allow patients to schedule
  their own appointments.

Develop a list of outliers – reasons that patients may take more time
– and add it to the scheduling notes so the front desk will know to
book long appointments.

By starting from the patient's point of view – the reason for calling
– you can build in a phone triage system that helps your staff ask

meaningful questions and schedule patients for the appropriate amounts of time. However, remember the more rules, the more mistakes – keep it simple.

Open-access scheduling

Determine your scheduling philosophy. Open access is a system of patient scheduling that allows any type of patient to be seen at any time of day, and we believe it is one of the most efficient ways to schedule today. There are two major advantages in moving to a more open-access system: physicians' ability to see their own patients and elimination of long patient waiting times – and therefore a reduction in patient complaints.

In open access, patients are scheduled according to the amount of time needed rather than the type of patient – don't restrict your schedule. For example, a physician might allow a "new-patient" slot at 9 a.m. only. This creates a barrier to new patient access. In general, these arbitrary appointment requirements clog the system and cause otherwise revenue-producing schedule slots to go unfilled – and frustrate patients. The one exception is a practice that is dependent on referrals. Referred patients need to be seen quickly.

An open schedule does not assign types of patients to certain times of day and experience shows that a more open, patient-focused scheduling system is better than a restricted one. Just remember to match the appointment time to the physician's style. In this way, you accept any patient any time, regardless of the reason, as long as the available time matches the anticipated length of services, and if you can accommodate them on the day they call or want to be seen, you will delight your patient.

The very act of developing this appointment system is a team-building exercise and the result, a well-designed appointment scheduling system, will render rewards in efficiency and will enhance productivity for both physicians and support staff. Most scheduling systems result in long patient waits, both for an appointment and for the exam. This one will not.

Let patients schedule their own appointments

As we can use rules to help staff schedule appropriately, scheduling rules can also work for patients. Patients can determine how long an appointment they need. Research shows that when patients know they get an appointment when they want it, they want less physician time. Patients who schedule their own appointments are likely to be respectful of the physician's time, seeing the physician's respect for the patient.

Prepare for appointments in a systematic way

Physicians need all pertinent information available at the time of the visit, so support staff need to begin pulling charts several days prior to the appointment. If a patient is coming from another facility, make sure outside records arrive before the appointment day. The day before the visit, support staff should review the medical records of the patients scheduled the next day to assure completeness and accuracy. Everything should be up to date. The physician should never have to leave an exam room to retrieve missing medical record information.

With the EHR, the health record will always be up to date and at the fingertips of your physicians.

Keep all exam rooms well-stocked

Stock each exam room appropriately, so that each physician can complete an entire visit without leaving the room. Stock all exam rooms identically, including the placement and organization of patient-education materials, so that a physician does not spend time fumbling through cabinets. Physicians should agree on what supplies, equipment and educational materials to place in all rooms. This uniformity saves money, keeps supplies current, simplifies exam room stocking and allows physicians the flexibility of using any room in the area.

> KEY: Stock every exam room at least daily.

Incorporating an EHR eliminates the need to stock educational material. At the click of mouse, you can generate any educational information necessary for each patient and he or she can walk out of the office with material in hand.

Develop protocols for rooming patients

Develop protocols for greeting patients, taking vital signs, gathering other important information (such as allergies) and writing down the presenting complaint.

Protocols should answer questions, such as: Does this patient need to:

■■ Have blood pressure taken?
■■ Have weight checked?
■■ Be dressed in a gown? or
■■ Complete any forms prior to the physician's arrival?

The rooming criteria chart is helpful both in training new staff and reminding existing staff of how you want your patients roomed.

Clearly, each staff member will bring his or her own personality and interpretation to this task, but it is vital to emphasize that this initial contact with the patient establishes the tone of the visit.

Use visit time wisely

Treat patients with respect, call them by name and make them feel as if you hear and care about their complaints. Give the patient information on why you request information or tests, and help them understand what to expect when they see the physician. Help the patients focus on the true reason for needing to see the physician. Patients are often vague and waste a great deal of the physician's time getting to the real problem.

This proactive, courteous, professional yet friendly approach to rooming a patient is a key factor in patient satisfaction and improved physician efficiency.

FIGURE 9.4 Rooming Criteria Chart

ROOMING CRITERIA

Reason For Visit	HT.	WT.	Head Circ	BP.	Temp	Pulse	Resp	Vision	Gown	Expose Area	Expose Feet	Ck Allergies	Ck Phone #	Health Maintenance Forms	Immunization Forms	Diabetic Flow Sheet	Chaperone
New CPE (includes P/P & Annuals)	X	X		X	X	X	X		After Prov sees			X	X	X	X		X
Est. CPE (includes P/P & Annuals)	X	X		X	X	X	X		X			X	X	X	X		X
School/Sports PE	X	X		X	X	X	X	X	X			X	X	X	X		X
WCC	X	X			X	X	X		X			X	X		X		
Chief Complaint				X	X					X		X	X	X	X		
ADULT																	
Pain any system				X	X	X				X		X	X	X	X		
Respiratory		X		X	X	X	X					X	X	X	X		
Cardiac		X		X	X	X	X		X			X	X	X	X		
Dermatology				X	X					X		X	X	X	X		
Orthopedic				X	X					X		X	X	X	X		
Diabetic		X		X							X	X	X	X	X	X	
CHILDREN	X	X	<18 m	3 y+	X	X	X	5 y+		X		X	X	X	X		
OMT				X								X	X	X	X		
Re checks (depends on reason for recheck use above criteria)																	
Repeat Pap		X		X	X				X				X				X
Breast Ck		X		X	X				X				X				X
Follow- up < 3 wks			X										X				
Lab Only													X				

When taking a BP be sure to watch to see if the monometer reading returns to zero.

When weighing a patient be sure to zero the scale first.

Staff to document Reason for Visit - Providers to obtain history.

Nurses rooming the patient can complete the medical, social and family histories before the physician enters the room; they can complete the review of systems and document vital signs. EHRs allow staff to collect information for physicians so they can better use their time.

Outline steps for discharging patients

Equally important to rooming a patient is a smooth, friendly and efficient discharge. Discharging is how we deal with treatment orders and follow-up plans after the physician sees the patient.

Patient discharge generates the tools for follow up. The order sheet system includes potential tests, pertinent educational materials, required referrals and follow-up needs – all of which can be automated and foolproof on an EHR – and completed while you are in the room with the patient. You no longer have to worry as to whether the work was completed.

Typically, the test verification form has been the order sheet. Once the order is executed, the staff place the order sheet in a tickler file for test verification and follow up; test verification checks to see that all tests ordered were completed and results returned to the office. When test results return, they are checked off the order sheet to complete the test verification task. The order sheet also tells support staff how to notify the patient of the results. Physicians usually want to review test results when they come back, but when used appropriately, the order sheet eliminates the physician's involvement for normal test results.

Today the EHR can eliminate this manual, time-consuming system. When the physician first accesses the EHR at the beginning of the work day, he or she will see a task list that holds all test results from the previous day. All the physician needs to do is review and forward results to the patient, with a note if appropriate. Then, with the push of a button everything is automatically filed in the EHR. In the past, physicians would hope they saw all the lab results they were supposed to see and that any abnormal results were identified.

In reality, many tests fell through the cracks. Often groups relied on patients to call the practice if they had not heard about their lab results (this does not reassure patients that you are actively involved in their care). This process alone will add an immeasurably higher level of safety to your practice, and patients will be delighted to receive timely results with physician comments and suggestions on literature to read or treatment plans.

With the EHR, the staff and the patient all know which actions the physician's instructions should trigger as the appointment concludes, the physician can print off a copy of the encounter along with any instructions, treatment plans and educational material, and the patient never needs to stop at the check-out desk. Again, this saves valuable resource time.

Document promptly after each patient

After each patient visit, the physician should promptly complete these tasks:

- ■■ Finish any dictation (recording the information is five times faster than writing it out);

- ■■ Complete the charge ticket and any necessary billing documentation;

- ■■ Check the message clipboard for any ASAP messages (see details on message handling under "Win the battle over paperwork"); and

- ■■ Review the chart for the next appointment.

You can automate these tasks. Using voice recognition or the point-and-click method, providers can document as they go. The system will automatically code as per the documentation, assuring accurate coding. While the EHR system automatically sends the bill, the physician can review the summary page for the next patient. Now you won't need to look for superbills at the end of the day. Imagine the hours of rework time eliminated when the system accounts for all charges and activates immediately to reduce the time between visit and payment.

In the midst of the patient care, there are two important, ongoing functions that play an important role in any efficient practice; paperwork and handling the telephones. Both deserve a plan.

Win the battle over paperwork

Delayed paperwork causes rework. Time drains from a practice when physicians must make multiple copies of an order, request or notice; or when staff members must field several telephone calls from a patient for one prescription buried in the bottom of an In box.

One solution is to educate support staff members to use a low-tech but effective system that assigns a priority to every piece of information before channeling it to physicians. This process keeps information moving smoothly throughout the day, from staff to physician and back to staff, without interrupting the physician or causing pileups.

With so much information flowing through a practice, a priority system is essential. An efficient system is as easy as providing every support staff member and physician with sheets of adhesive colored dots and three mailboxes, labeled In, Out, and Action. Also, place ASAP (as soon as possible) clipboards (or just clips), between the exam rooms.

Staff members triage information for physicians, sorting all paper, requests and messages into a hierarchy of priorities. To minimize interruptions, have staff members put questions in writing.

The In box. The In box is for all other paperwork that the physician needs or asks to see. Encourage physicians to empty all In boxes each Friday to avoid a monumental task in the future. Many physicians spend Saturday cleaning out their In boxes and are amazed at what they find.

The Out box. Have support staff empty the Out box hourly. As physicians act on ASAP and action items during the course of the day, they place them in their Out box. As part of the workflow, whoever rooms patients also empties Out boxes. Even though this seems basic, emptying Out boxes is one of the hardest things for staff members to remember. Marked with color-coded dots, these papers and messages take the support staff a matter of seconds to dispatch. They include items needing only a signature, schedule changes or urgent notes (The registered nurse should determine the urgency of medical messages).

The ASAP clip and Action boxes. Use ASAP clips for items that need an action completed between patients or for quick signatures. The rule is if it takes 10 seconds to act on the message, put it in the ASAP clip. This facilitates timely paper flow throughout the day. A good example is the prescription refill that only needs a quick signature, yet often ends up at the bottom of an In box, and the delay in responding to the message triggers several additional telephone calls. To help maintain good customer service, place patient information requests that may not be urgent but are easy to answer quickly in the ASAP clip.

Use the Action box for all items that need resolution before the end of the day.

While this system works well, automating the process will save enormous amounts of time for the staff and physicians. One of the major reasons for moving to an electronic system is to decrease paper. So visualize the system above in an automated state. Messages come across via e-mail and providers can forward their messages with instructions or e-mail patients directly. Electronic messaging does not get lost, can easily be forwarded and access to the patient's record is at the click of the mouse.

Empower support staff to direct telephone and mail traffic and you will immediately improve practice efficiency.

Opening mail

From a productivity perspective, support staff should open the mail and respond to as much as they can, giving the physicians only what they need prioritized in the appropriate box.

Phone system – nurse calls

Have the person who can handle the call answer the call. Patients transferred to several different staff members before getting to someone who can actually answer their questions results in dissatisfaction. Consider a phone tree that sends scheduling calls to the scheduler, nurse calls to the nurse and billing calls to the billing department.

EHR benefits the practice by enabling patients to e-mail their questions or make their own appointments – you can respond without having to play phone tag and you will save resource time, which saves money for the practice.

Phone messages

Phone message forms can signal immediately the action required. Use different kinds of forms for telephone messages, prescriptions, personal calls, and one for patient encounters, with a duplicate that goes into a patient record.

All of these forms can go on your website for patients to fill out and e-mail back to your practice. An EHR system immediately files information into the electronic record without a staff member touching a phone message.

Put it in writing

Encourage staff to put questions and issues in writing to avoid interrupting physicians. Interruptions cause delays. Remember to develop systems that support efficiency and make the best use of a physician's time.

Follow-up is mandatory

Repeatedly, physicians say that they have a deep-seated fear that something may fall through the cracks – test results not communicated, a prescription not ordered as promised or misplaced documentation. This can lead to disgruntled – or sicker – patients and could even put the practice in legal jeopardy.

EHRs assure that precise, documented up-to-date information is always available, and makes things flow more smoothly, as well as guarantee that tasks are routinely completed.

Keep a master calendar of all mandatory meetings, days working in other locations and any other non-daily activity in the physician's schedule. This helps prevent forgetting to add a meeting to the schedule and mis-scheduling patients, which frustrates physicians, inconveniences the patient, and creates a great deal of staff rework, which is very costly. One last comment about rescheduling patients – they hate it and may use it as a reason to find another physician. Plan ahead. Set up effective systems that will help to alleviate the need to reschedule patients.

Systems check lists

A good patient-flow system should include:

- ■■ Greeting;
- ■■ Visit prep;
- ■■ Room stocking;
- ■■ Rooming criteria;
- ■■ Order execution; and
- ■■ Follow-up.

An efficient communication system should include:

- ■■ In, Out, and Action boxes for the physician and ASAP clips between exam rooms;
- ■■ Message identification, prioritization and flow systems;
- ■■ Tickler systems for patient communication, including reporting test results, scheduling appointments and sending reminders of services needed;
- ■■ Tracking services and charges so billing can occur in a timely, accurate manner; and

■■ Telephone protocols that use a registered nurse to triage patients' medical calls.

Whether manual or automated systems are in place, addressing each area will help to ensure an efficient and productive operation.

Don't forget the housekeeping, storage and stocking tasks. While not automated, they are essential for an efficient practice. Keep adequate supplies on hand and all exam rooms well-stocked with supplies in identical places from room to room.

CHAPTER 10

PRINCIPLE V
Distributing Tasks Appropriately

THE FIRST STEP IN DISTRIBUTING TASKS APPROPRIATELY is to identify the scope of practice for each position.

The scope of practice relates to all tasks that each position is allowed to do by state law or regulations. In most states medical assistants work under the physicians' license and are managed by nurses. However, in other states, registered nurses cannot supervise medical assistants. It is important that you know the limitations in your state. Put together a matrix, as shown in Figure 10.1, which clearly shows the limitation of each position.

Job descriptions for health care practitioners and support staff

To work at optimal efficiency, a practice needs qualified people doing appropriate tasks within appropriate time frames.

An easy way to identify current tasks is by using the Statement of Duties tool as shown in Figure 10.2, which provides an organized format for obtaining employees' and practitioners' impressions of what tasks they are

FIGURE 10.1 **Ambulatory Clinic's Scope of Practice by Category**

	Front Office Staff	Medical Assistant	Licensed Practical Nurse	Registered Nurse
Credentials	None	Graduate of accredited school	LPN license; bi-annual renewal	RN license; bi-annual renewal
Limitations				
Scope of practice				

Medications:
  Oral
  Subcutaneous
  Intradermal
  Intramuscular
  Intravenous
  Inhaled				

IV Therapy:
  IV insert/DC
  IV fluid admin
  IV drug admin				

Phlebotomy				
12 Lead EKG				
Small volume nebulizers				
Pulse oximetry				
Feeding tubes				
Telephone triage				
Patient assessment				
Patient visits				
Medication refills				
Rooming criteria				
Follow-up				

doing in their present positions. Each employee and practitioner needs to complete this form in the following way:

1. Enter the employee or practitioner's name, job title, department name and date.

2. Identify this position's key process – the purpose for hiring the person. The key process is what you will measure when determining the work volume of each position; it's usually the key volume indicator. The key process differs from the job title in that it explains what process the employee is actually doing – you hire a receptionist, the job title is receptionist, but the actual task is to check in patients. The title is not clear enough to establish a key volume indicator.

3. Identify the key volume indicator. This drives work volume. The number of patient appointments drives the volume of work for the receptionist.

4. Have each practitioner and employee list each of the tasks they perform, and whether they do the task on a daily, weekly, monthly or yearly basis.

5. Estimate the number of times the employee completes the task on a weekly basis.

6. Document the method for counting each task. For example, the receptionist checks in patients – count each patient checked in for an appointment.

7. Determine the most appropriate skill level to perform the task. It is important to identify each job classification's scope of practice, to assure appropriate use of different types of employees. This varies from state to state.

The Statement of Duties form is a key tool when analyzing your practice. It is helpful to use a patient's visit through the office as a tool for categorizing the tasks associated with an appointment. The categories include triaging, scheduling, obtaining medical records, admitting, rooming, diagnosing and treating, teaching, discharging, following up and billing.

FIGURE 10.2 **Statement of Duties Tool**

STATEMENT OF DUTIES

Name: Jane Doe   Department: Family Medicine

Title: Receptionist   Key volume indicator: Patients seen

Key process: Prepare charts and patient check in   Date: 6/05

TASK	VOLUME PER WEEK	HOW COUNTED	SKILL LEVEL
Check in charts	500	Each chart	Clerical – low
Prepare charts	500	Each chart	Clerical – low
Check in patients	480	Patients seen	Receptionist – moderate

How do you create a job description?

Within each of the tasks required as a patient moves through the system, list everything that needs to happen to make that part of the visit go smoothly. Determine who on the team – clerk, medical assistant or registered nurse – has the appropriate skill level to carry out the task.

Once each employee completes his or her form, you should know all the work associated with each patient as well as tasks performed that do not relate to the patient visit. You also will have a list of the appropriate skill levels for each task. With this information, you can determine the most appropriate employee to perform each task. The next step is to develop job descriptions.

To identify the actual number of employees you need in each job, conduct a time study for each task. The more repetitive and consistent the task, the less number of samples you need to know if the time is valid and reliable. If the task times vary considerably, you will need a larger time sample.

By using the identified task time multiplied by an estimated number of appointments you anticipate each day, you can determine how much time each of these tasks will take and how many employees of each skill level you will need in your practice.

Finally, besides the tasks that are driven by the number of patients you see, there is ongoing work that needs to be done regardless of your patient volume. These fixed tasks include such things as opening and sorting mail, stocking exam rooms and providing reception and phone coverage.

Identify the time needed per day to perform each task and allocate an average time per day for these tasks. You can identify the number of employees you need to staff both the phones and the reception desk by determining the volume of work per day. Remember, you must minimally staff these positions based on the hours of operation. If the time study shows you need five hours of receptionist time to do the tasks you have assigned that job and the clinic is open eight hours per day, you must staff the reception desk eight hours each day and try to bring other tasks to the receptionist that s/he can do when not checking in patients.

By defining the roles, responsibilities and appropriate skill levels required for each staff person's job, you have taken another step towards building an effective medical practice.

Evaluating employee performance

It is always helpful to review the job description as you give an evaluation, to remind the employee of the position's expectations at your organization. It is not fair to an employee to be evaluated on tasks that are outside their scope of practice or that are not included in their job description. Evaluation is a wonderful time to reward employees for a job well done – their success is your success.

Look at the physician's time

What should a physician do? How should he or she spend time in the office? Or, perhaps more important, what should a physician avoid doing? Observations over the years show us that in the most productive and profitable practices, physicians confine the majority of their time to these key tasks:

■■ Reviewing medical records;

■■ Conducting medical exams and performing procedures;

■■ Developing and communicating treatment plans;

■■ Documenting information, treatment plans and services;

■■ Communicating with patients' families or significant others;

■■ Reviewing tests results; and

■■ Coding charge tickets.

Physicians who routinely spend time on other tasks may be unintentionally wasting time. The litmus test of an activity that justifies a physician's time is this:

"Is this a task that someone else could safely, legally and effectively complete?"

If the answer is yes, then the physician should not routinely do that task. We need to learn to leverage physician time much as dentists do – dentists use support staff far better than physicians do. Dentists go in the exam room when only a dentist can do the work; otherwise, either the hygienist or the assistant does the work.

What should a registered nurse do?

A registered nurse is a great asset to any practice when used appropriately and a great expense when used inappropriately. The key is their ability to work within the RN scope of practice and perform independent activities. One example is telephone triage: If the major responsibility of the triage nurse is teaching, the position becomes a value-added position. However, if you require the physician to review every call, then a lower-skill-level employee can better handle the task. If the triage nurse is simply a "gate keeper," patients will find a way to access the system by either going to the ER or urgent care center or calling another physician. Develop an open-access system to save resource time and delight your patients. Understand the purpose for having an RN.

Constant interruptions dramatically slow down a practice. Allowing a nurse to handle daily phone calls will increase physician productivity. Our research shows that a registered nurse can save a physician up to two hours a day by handling all the patient problem telephone calls. You can easily accomplish this with written protocols.

Patient education is another excellent task for a registered nurse. While education is extremely important, it also is very time consuming for the physician. Allowing your registered nurse to conduct patient education will also free up the physician to see more patients in the office.

You also can delegate to your registered nurse such tasks as minor procedures and patient assessments.

Remember, clerical support staff should complete most of the clerical work.

Distributing tasks appropriately and delegating tasks to the lowest-skill-level person that can perform the task safely and legally is a good business move, and more important, it will improve morale. When both employees and physicians are working at their potential, they are better able to focus on patient care.

What should a licensed practical nurse do?

Training for licensed practical nurses (LPNs) tends to be more task oriented: LPNs are usually able to draw blood, give medications, assist with procedures, and recognize and meet basic patient needs. LPNs are not trained to make nursing diagnoses and treatment plans. Triage is not the best role for most LPNs because their training is not in assessment.

What should a medical assistant do?

The medical assistant usually works under the license of the physician. In reality, a medical assistant in a private practice can perform any task the physician trains her/him for; however, it is best to check with your professional liability provider, as well as the State Board of Medicine for their opinion on the appropriate scope of practice.

What should a nonphysician provider do?

Nonphysician providers have an important role in medicine today; they may help bridge the gap created by the looming physician shortage. However, it is important to understand the nonphysician provider's role in your practice; as dentists do with hygienists, identify exactly the role for each nonphysician provider in your practice. It is not helpful when nonphysician providers compete with physicians for patients: if patient overflow goes to the nonphysician provider when the physician's schedule is full, the nonphysician provider will be seeing patients beyond their scope of practice and must rely on the physician for back up. This is neither satisfying for the patient nor the nonphysician provider, and can be very frustrating for the physician (who is already behind). Nonphysician providers are invaluable when performing the appropriate duties.

Take the time to understand the scope of practice for each team member. Distribute tasks according to skill level and you will have a more satisfied staff. Staff members doing appropriate tasks function together to provide quality patient care – that's medical teamwork at its best.

CHAPTER 11

PRINCIPLE VI

Creating an Interdependent Team

Teamwork

Coming together is a beginning;

Keeping together is progress;

Working together is success.

—Henry Ford

THE KEY TO ANY WELL-FUNCTIONING MEDICAL PRACTICE is teamwork. Patients expect the same quality of care each time they come to the office; the efficient practice develops systems that allow for continuity of care when either the physician or the support staff is out of the office.

Each practice must determine what the "team" looks like in their practice. In a solo practice, obviously the team is the entire office, but in a large group practice, it is harder to define the team. To determine who should be on your team, consider:

- ■■ With whom the patient interacts and how you can be assured that the patient will receive consistent, timely information with each interaction; and

■■ Who will step in when one of the usual staff is out of the office? Often, teams consist of more than one physician with shared staff to assure that when a staff member is out someone else knows the practice.

When forming a team and outlining roles, clearly define and agree upon expectations and desired outcomes – the practice will function like a winning football team. The coach reviews the play with the entire team so that every player knows his or her position and action, then the team executes the play together to score. Sometimes players must leave their positions to make a play in a teammate's absence. To make this happen, everyone needs to agree on the team definition.

FIRST, recognize that it is probably impractical for every physician to have his or her own exclusive support staff. One-on-one staffing is not efficient unless you move all deskwork to the front office, and research shows that moving more tasks closer to the physician is most efficient.

SECOND, establish uniform systems, routines and ongoing communication plans. This is critical to serving several physicians. Remember Principle IV: Decreasing Unnecessary Variation.

THIRD, construct each position carefully to include responsibilities that use each position's expertise and value each position equally. Do not show favoritism; your practice cannot run smoothly without everyone on the team participating. The receptionists and schedulers are as important to the efficiency of your practice as your nurse is – but seldom do they feel as valued. You must give your entire team a sense of purpose, control and realistic expectations.

You can further guide your team by clearly communicating the practice's mission statement, as we discussed in Chapter 4. A mission statement outlines the practice philosophy. Place this statement where it is visible to both staff members and patients.

To help the team function as a single unit, you must also develop communication tools.

Communication tools

We recommend three communication tools for every practice that does not use an EHR and we will discuss those first. Then, we will illustrate the differences with EHR communications.

TOOL 1: Appointment schedule. Manual schedules are nearly useless as a communication tool. Only the front desk knows about schedule changes and unless you make a new copy hourly, they are quickly outdated. This is also true with a computer system only accessed by the front desk.

Do not view the schedule as a tool for scheduling only. View it as a communication tool that allows the scheduler to communicate with the physician and nursing staff. The two major elements, as shown in Figure 11.1, are time as reflected in appointment type and remarks.

The Appointment Type is a clue to the length of time the visit requires and helps the office staff plan the day – remembering that the schedule is only a tool and not an absolute. If a patient is late and another patient has arrived, room the early patient. Do not wait for the late patient, keep the patient flow moving. Many offices that run on time bring patents back to the exam room as they arrive. Few patients, even if they are roomed out of order, wait very long when a practice runs on time.

FIGURE 11.1 **Scheduling Tool**

NAME	PT. #	AGE	APPOINTMENT TYPE	REMARKS
John Doe	1234546	45	Con	Miller/OSR/4/94/diabetic
Jane Doe	654321	22	BV	BO#!/sore throat/3 days
Sue Smith	456123	35	New	NPE/3/91/no problem
Bill Jones	123654	55	EV	RPE/4/93/diabetic

The Remarks column in Figure 11.1 holds the most valuable information. Use this area to show what information needs to be ready for the visit as well as how to prepare the exam room.

TOOL 2: Patient visit worksheet. The second tool is the patient visit worksheet (see Figure 11.2). This tool communicates information to the physician when using a manual system. Your staff will use this tool three different ways.

First, your support staff members use the tool during visit prep to record any missing information, whether outside records have arrived, allergies, medications, and so on.

FIGURE 11.2 **Patient Visit Worksheet**

PATIENT VISIT WORKSHEET

Patient name: Clinic:

Daytime phone: Personal physician:

Reason for visit:

New – complete 1,2,4,5   BV – complete 1,4,5

Con – complete 1,2,3,4,5   EV – complete 1,2,4,5

---

1. Vital signs: Ht   WT   BP   Temp   LMP

---

2. Recent tests: Labs   EKG   Mammogram   Treadmill   Echo
                       Procto   Other X-rays

---

3. Outside records: films records

---

4. Medications name   dose   last refill   last appointment

---

5. Allergies   .

Notes:

Next, staff members use the tool during rooming. The person rooming the patient sees the appointment type annotation and knows exactly what kind of information he or she must gather.

Finally, physicians use this form to take notes for dictation purposes while talking with patients. This is not part of the medical record, so it will remain in the worksheet until the transcriptionist completes the dictation. By dictating from this form, physicians are able to dictate all essential information, including information the support staff usually write in the medical record.

Using an EHR completely eliminates the manual system. Each chief complaint or reason for the visit will have a corresponding template. Each template will identify the exact information needed for the visit. Information is entered only once and can be reviewed by all appropriate staff members and at each subsequent visit. The system will also cue the physician regarding the need for preventive medicine, prescription refills, and/or follow-up treatment. All test results will be in the computerized record so you will never need to look for missing information.

TOOL 3: Patient visit order sheet. The third tool we use is a patient visit order sheet (see Figure 11.3). You will put your practice at risk by missing abnormal test results without systems to assure that test verification and results reporting are completed in a timely manner. Physicians use this tool to communicate with their patients and then the staff. An order sheet provides you the opportunity to review the orders with the patient and give them a copy to take with them. Patients appreciate having a written copy of their orders, because they do not have to try to remember everything.

The original copy goes to the staff for processing. This way, physicians do not have to wait until they are off the phone to give verbal orders. This will significantly reduce mistakes as well as time.

Use this form for order verification. Place this form in a tickler file until all orders are completed. The tickler file allows your staff to follow up on all outstanding orders.

FIGURE 11.3 **Patient Visit Order Sheet**

PATIENT VISIT ORDER SHEET

Patient name: Physician:

Daytime phone:

Test Results: Special needs:

(how to inform patient of test results)   Outside records

Call patient   Financial counseling

Form letter

Dictated letter

Date reported

Visit follow-up

(appointment category and time frame)

BV   EV   with:

Tests:

(list the most common tests ordered)   Stat   Routine   ICD-9

Lab:

Radiology:

Cardiology:

Health maintenance:

Educational materials:

Nursing instructions:

The last purpose for this form is to communicate physician desires for patient education and follow-up.

While this form is better than no form, it is still a manual system and is only as good as the staff that monitors the tickler file. The only foolproof system is the EHR – if there is one reason to invest in the EHR, it is the order entry system. No longer will you worry about what fell through the cracks: when you order a test and the results are not in your system the next morning, an alert appears on your desktop. Eliminating the time (often overtime) it takes staff to order tests, monitor results, and notify patients will save many hours of labor.

In addition to the hard tools just presented, here are some intangible tools for your team.

Weekly meetings

Conduct short weekly meetings to improve communication within the practice and begin to learn what does and does not go well. Many groups choose one day a week to have lunch together and talk about how to improve service to patients. Informal environments help make all players feel relaxed and comfortable – team building at its best! No white coats or name badges at the meetings, please! Encourage staff to be themselves, Bob, Mary, Kathleen, etc.

At these weekly meetings, value each person equally for insight, suggestions and ideas. This will empower staff to work on ways to improve support to the physician/patient interaction and improve value as perceived by the patient.

In addition to weekly meetings, the group should meet for five minutes each morning to examine daily operational issues.

The role of the morning huddle

How do you keep the sense of teamwork and interdependency going once the practice is running? Schedule a daily huddle – a short, informal meeting of the physicians and support staff first thing in the morning. The purpose of this meeting is to proactively plan the day's activities. Include:

- **Old business**: Review yesterday's schedule. This is very helpful for new support staff. Review the good and the bad. Identify key patients for follow-up calls to check on their progress (this is a major patient pleaser).

■■ **New business**: Review today's schedule for issues that are likely to arise: patients with unusual needs, special tests that may be required, staffing issues that everyone should know about. This is an ideal time to communicate how the physician would like the staff to handle same-day, urgent patients. By communicating this early in the day, your support staff will not have to interrupt you to ask you where and when to add patients.

■■ **Future business**: Review tomorrow's schedule. Look for scheduling problems that could cause havoc tomorrow. This will give you time to fix the problems and a chance to prepare for tomorrow. This is a good time to identify and call chronic no-show patients, or people who are always late.

Unique clinic issues

In many clinics, there likely is another element of the team: administrative staff members.

It is just as important to keep the lines of communication open with administration as it is between your physicians and staff. This open communication will lead to a sense of partnership and teamwork.

Unfortunately, this communication does not always happen. Administrators and physicians can find themselves at odds with each other. Administrators press management to decrease operational expenses and physicians to increase productivity. This results in tremendous frustration for both physicians and management.

It is essentially a matter of focus: administrators are interested in cutting expenses and ask physicians to increase revenues. Change the dynamics. Have both physicians and administrators responsible for both revenues and expenses. Working together toward common goals and implementation plans assures that administrators and physicians both feel successful.

Keeping costs in line and patient counts up are both necessary for a successful practice. It is counterproductive when administrators implement a plan that decreases costs without understanding the impact on physician abilities to increase revenues. The answer comes from collaboration, not conflict.

A well-defined mission statement with agreed-upon attainable goals sets the framework for the practice. Clear, concise communication among all team members including staff, physicians and administrators assures success.

Teams are not alike, and work volume varies by team for many reasons. It is not as important that they are different as it is that you allocate resources by the volume of work.

CHAPTER 12

PRINCIPLE VII

Allocating Resources by Volume of Work

RESOURCE ALLOCATION IS A HOT TOPIC in group practices today. Historically, groups allocated resources by discipline. For example, a physician's allotment may be one office, two exam rooms and one office assistant. A physician's assistant received less, one shared office, one exam room and no support staff. Hierarchy dictated resource allocation.

Today, we allocate resources differently. We now realize that work volume is the key to resource allocation. Physicians who see high daily patient volumes need more support staff and more space to maximize productivity.

We also realize that nonphysician providers need support that is commensurate to their work volume. Just because they are not physicians does not mean they do not generate a great deal of work.

Patient-visit volume is one measurement you can use to determine support staff and space needs. Patient visits generate most but not all of the clinic's work.

Space and resources are becoming more expensive. One way to combat this increase is to better utilize both support staff and space. We already discussed the advantages of using team staffing; consider also sharing exam rooms.

The exercise you performed in Chapter 4 can be used to effectively share exam room space: Hang a form on the outside of each exam room. Each time you put a patient in an exam room, record the time. When the patient leaves the room, again record the time. Subtract the time out from the time in to establish the room utilization time for each patient. Compile all the times each day for several weeks. You will be amazed at the small percentage of time each exam room is actually used.

Creative master schedules

This brings us back to the concept of master schedules. Often times you can add another physician without adding space if you become creative and stagger or expand hours. This increases physician availability, a plus for patients. By extending the hours, you can better meet your patients' needs. Before and after work are popular appointment times for working patients. The lunch hour also is popular (lunch hour works only when the physician is running on time). Senior citizens seem to prefer daylight hours. Working the usual 9 a.m. to noon and 2 p.m. to 5 p.m. may hinder the physician's ability to maintain an adequate patient base.

Allocating resources by volume of work will allow you to better manage expenses, resulting in a decreased cost per visit.

Wasted space

Analyze non-revenue-generating space. Is your waiting room too large? As your practice begins to run on time, you will no longer need a large waiting room. Some practices eliminate the waiting room all together and have a greeter meet the patient as they arrive and take them to an exam room for check-in, eliminating non-revenue-generating space and one wait for the patient.

Office space is another example of non-revenue-generating space. Many groups are moving to physician-shared office space. Some use cubicles in a large room; others have offices in another area and only a small workspace in the clinic. Still others no longer feel they need an office on site since each exam room has a computer and documentation occurs in the exam room during each patient visit.

There are many solutions to space constraints. Remember space is normally the second major expense after labor. Poor space utilization is costly to a practice.

When looking at resources, focus on revenue-generating activities. With electronic communication, no longer do you have to house non-revenue-generating activities in high-cost space – using prime space for transcription, billing and collection activities can be expensive, and with technology, many of these functions are done outside the clinic entirely.

Now that you have an understanding of the 7 Guiding Principles of practice management, let us look at a smooth-running medical practice that embraces all of these principles in a manual system, and then learn how the tech-savvy practice can benefit from the EHR.

CHAPTER 13 | **A Smooth Operation**

WHEN WE LEFT ANN ACKNEY AT THE END OF CHAPTER 2, she had lost all confidence in Dr. Frazzle. She has begun seeing Dr. Smooth.

It is Monday morning and Ms. Ackney calls Dr. Smooth's office for an appointment. Mary, the receptionist, courteously answers the phone and asks Ann pertinent questions to learn the reason for the appointment and further information that will allow her to schedule Ann for the correct amount of time. Patient-focused scheduling enables Mary to find time in the schedule for Ann. Mary schedules Ann for Wednesday at 4:30 p.m. Mary also verifies Ann's demographic information, to ensure that the Medical Records Department pulls the correct chart and reviews Ann's co-pay responsibility. This will eliminate patient embarrassment or surprise at the time of the appointment. The Medical Records Department automatically pulls Ms. Ackney's chart and sends it to Dr. Smooth's office.

On Tuesday afternoon, Betty, the registered nurse for Dr. Smooth and his partner, prepares charts for the next day. She pulls Ann's chart and quickly scans it for accuracy and completeness. She assesses preparation needs for the visit. Betty notices that Ms. Ackney's last mammogram report is not in the chart, so Betty pulls the results up on the computer, prints it and places it on the chart for the physician.

Wednesday morning, Suzy, the other support staff person, takes a quick inventory of all exam rooms and stocks them. Stocking exam rooms identically makes it faster and easier for Suzy to restock. When Dr. Smooth arrives at the clinic Wednesday, Suzy reviews yesterday's, today's and tomorrow's schedules with him. Because Suzy is new to the practice, they review yesterday's schedule to learn how they can work better together. Dr. Smooth also notes that two of his patients from yesterday could use a personal call from Nurse Betty to follow up on their conditions.

As Dr. Smooth reviews today's schedule, he notes that one of the patients on his schedule was admitted to the hospital last night. Suzy cancels the appointment, allowing time to schedule another patient. Dr. Smooth also notes his 1 p.m. patient often forgets appointments and asks Suzy to call him.

As Dr. Smooth looks over tomorrow's schedule, he notes an error. Correcting it today prevents confusion tomorrow and saves time. Reacting to a problem always takes more time than planning. This entire process took less than five minutes, yet it alleviated confusion, a potentially missed appointment and inappropriate appointments, and it facilitated appropriate follow-up on patients.

On Wednesday at 4:30 p.m., Ms. Ackney arrives and Mary greets her warmly. Ann notes that there are no glass windows separating her from the receptionist. It feels much friendlier than Dr. Frazzle's office. After a quick check-in and payment of her co-pay, Ms. Ackney takes a seat in the clean, neat waiting room. Within five minutes, Suzy calls her by name and the two walk to the exam room. On the way, Suzy verifies Ms. Ackney's address and phone number to facilitate timely follow-up.

Because Ms. Ackney is in today for a chief complaint, Suzy takes her vital signs, identifies the medications she is presently taking and asks if she needs any refills. Suzy also asks about allergies, symptoms and duration of her chief complaint. Suzy completes part of the prescription for the medication Ann requests. She then records the information on the visit prep sheet and places it on the front of the chart. After instructing Ann to change into a gown, Suzy leaves the room, places the chart outside the door and marks the room number on the schedule hanging on Dr. Smooth's office door.

Five minutes later, Dr. Smooth completes dictating the last patient's chart and notes on his schedule that Ann is ready in Room 22. Before Dr. Smooth enters the exam room, he sees a message on the ASAP clip between exam rooms. He quickly glances at the message, noting it only needs a signature. After Dr. Smooth signs the message and drops it in the Out box, he reviews Ann's visit prep and summary sheets on the front of her chart. This takes less than two minutes.

Dr. Smooth walks into the room and greets Ms. Ackney. He reviews her history with her and notes that the chart is accurate and complete. After concluding that Ann indeed needs the medication she is requesting, Dr. Smooth adjusts the dosage and signs the prescription Suzy prepared.

He decides to do a small procedure and finds everything he needs is in the correct place. When he completes the exam, Dr. Smooth reviews the orders with Ann, discusses how Betty will call her tomorrow with the test results and hands Ann her prescription. Dr. Smooth then asks if she has any other questions. Ann feels relieved (and cared for) by the attention Dr. Smooth shows her and feels he is extremely competent, thorough and informative. She has no other questions. As Dr. Smooth leaves the exam room, he instructs Ms. Ackney to talk to Betty before she leaves the office.

When he walks back to his office to dictate, he hands Betty the order sheet. On the order sheet, he requests educational materials for Ann and asks Betty to review the information with Ann before she leaves the office. He completes his dictation and moves on to his last patient of the day.

Once Dr. Smooth finishes seeing his last patient, he returns to his office, dictates the last chart and prepares to leave. He glances in his Action box and notes two forms to sign. Suzy placed all action items in the Action box with the appropriate back-up material attached. Because all the information he needs is available, he reviews each item and signs both. He then places them in his Out box. He also quickly reviews the messages the nurse responded to today. Betty handled all calls appropriately; however, Dr. Smooth feels one of the calls needs follow-up tomorrow. He quickly jots a note to the nurse, places it in his Out box and is off to make rounds at the hospital.

It was another rewarding day for Dr. Smooth. He was able to care for 25 patients and still left on time. He completed all the charge tickets for both the hospital and clinic visits for the day and sent them to the billing office.

Meanwhile, Betty greets Ms. Ackney as she walks out of the exam room. Betty gives her some educational material and reviews it with her before she leaves. She also reviews the orders and gives Ann a copy to take with her in case she forgets what Dr. Smooth ordered. She then asks if Ann has any questions. Betty instructs Ann to stop by the lab on her way out of the clinic. They discuss an appropriate time for Betty to call with the results. Betty notes the time on the order sheet and places a copy of the order sheet in her tickler file.

The lab information is on the computer when Betty arrives at work Thursday morning. The lab values are slightly elevated; however, Betty knows from the prewritten orders how to handle the situation. At 1 p.m., Betty calls Ms. Ackney to give her the lab test results and explain the care plan. She documents her conversation with Ann. Dr. Smooth receives a copy of the documentation so he knows what transpired with his patient.

Ann is amazed when she receives a follow-up call from Betty on Friday, just to see how she is doing.

Dr. Smooth's efficient practice impresses Ann; the entire interaction seems to have run like clockwork. When friends or acquaintances mention they are looking for a physician, Ann does not hesitate to refer Dr. Smooth.

However, as costs continue to increase, Dr. Smooth finds the labor-intensive systems, while effective, very costly. His wife, also a physician, works in a group practice that is converting to the EHR. He believes that this is the next step in maintaining an efficient and cost-effective practice. He tries to envision what his practice would look like using an EHR and, luckily, is asked to join his wife's group.

Ms. Ackney's visits compared a chaotic practice to a smooth-running practice that uses the 7 Guiding Principles. Her next visit will illustrate how Dr. Smooth joined Dr. Tech-Savvy's practice, enhancing the 7 Guiding Principles by using an EHR.

CHAPTER 14 | # The Tech-Savvy Practice

ANN ACKNEY RECEIVES A LETTER IN THE MAIL from Dr. Smooth explaining his new affiliation with his wife's practice, which had recently converted to using an electronic health record. He invites her to access his new practice's website and explains that she would now have immediate access to his practice. The practice's new name: Tech-Savvy Physicians.

This intrigues Ann because she uses computers for communication, both at work and home.

Ann logs in to her computer and accesses the Tech-Savvy Physicians' website. It is friendly, easy to navigate and secure. Because this is a new system, it asks Ann to fill out demographic and insurance information, and review and sign the HIPAA (Health Insurance Portability and Accountability Act) forms. Then it asks her to complete social, family and medical history forms. She also fills out a form called "review of systems," which records problems in each of her body's systems (this is the form patients usually complete while sitting in the waiting room). She only needs to identify those areas of concern.

The next step on the site is to list her current medications. Because she does not have them in front of her, she stops, walks to the medicine cabinet, returns with all her medications, and proceeds to enter them into the system. It asks her to name her preferred pharmacy, which is printed on the medication container's label. It is very convenient and Ann knows they have the right information on file.

At the click of the mouse, Ann can access educational information. She also notices that when she needs an appointment she can schedule it herself. Her annual exam is due, so Ann decides to try her hand at the scheduling system.

As Ann clicks on the scheduling system, the scheduling rules pop up. It asks her for the reason for her visit as well as her provider of choice and when she would like the appointment. Ann can see that Dr. Smooth is booked for two weeks, but there's an opening to see one of Dr. Smooth's new partners, Dr. Samantha Tech-Savvy. Ann decides to see Dr. Tech-Savvy, so she fills in the information and her scheduling options appear. She chooses the time most convenient and after she makes the appointment, a screen appears with instructions on the tests that will be ordered as well as any medications that should be refilled. In addition, a map of the office's new location appears, with directions from her home. After she completes the task and exits the website, her e-mail message box blinks that she has a new message. A confirmation message has been sent to her in less than 10 seconds! It thanks her for scheduling her appointment, explaining that her mammogram was scheduled three days prior to her appointment and was pre-approved by her insurance company. Ann is thrilled.

When she scheduled the appointment, Ann requested a reminder e-mail 48 hours prior to her visit; one week later Ann receives the reminder e-mail regarding her 9:30 a.m. appointment on Friday. Ann is curious about this new office.

As Ann arrives at the clinic, Gayle greets her. Because this is Ann's first visit to Tech-Savvy Physicians, Gayle asks Ann if she can take her photo. Ann approves the digital photo, which is now part of her electronic record and Gayle walks Ann to the exam room. Once in the room, Gayle accesses Ann's records on the . She notes that

Ann's co-pay is $20. Gayle collects Ann's co-pay and enters the payment into the system. She reassures Ann that her insurance covers today's visit and that her insurance has already sent a confirmation of her coverage. Gayle reminds Ann that at the end of the visit she should receive a receipt showing her co-pay as paid. (Gayle wears a small, zipped pack around her waist to hold the money and follows proper accounting principles for cash controls by verifying her cash at the end of each day.)

When Ann made the appointment via the practice website, she noticed that she could pay for her visit on the website by credit card. If she'd entered all the necessary information at that time, she could show up for the appointment and all she'd need to do is electronically sign the payment.

Gayle verifies the reason for the visit and pulls up the appropriate visit template in the EHR computer system. She then follows the system's instructions regarding the information needed for that template. She also notes that Ann had updated all of her information only a week earlier and asks her how she liked inputting the information herself. Ann replied that it was easy, convenient and she really felt it was more accurate because she had time to check information and labels at home.

Gayle then asks Ann if she would prefer to change into a gown now or talk with the physician first. Ann absolutely hates to wait, so she knew that if she changed into a gown now, she'd only have to wait once instead of twice. Ann opts to change into a gown and Gayle steps out for a moment. She returns to the room to complete Ann's visit prep.

She weighs and measures Ann. When Ann steps on the scale in the exam room, the computer system automatically records the results of her weight and height in the EHR along with her BMI (body mass index). The same is true for her temperature, pulse, respiration and blood pressure. Because Ann had entered all her basic information in the record from home, Gayle had little to review. Gayle leaves the room assuring Ann that Dr. Tech-Savvy would be right in.

Ann is amazed that Tech-Savvy Physicians has no waiting room (where she'd be exposed to sick patients!). Things really were changing. She also noted at how few support staff she saw standing around. No longer was there a receptionist desk or medical records lying all over. She didn't have to go to a separate desk to pay her co-pay and no longer did several different staff members ask her the same questions. It feels so efficient.

In between patients, Dr. Tech-Savvy accesses her schedule at a workstation. She checks for any messages that can be handled easily and then glances at Ann's record prior to entering the exam room. She reviews Ann's photo and some personal information about her that she could use to break the ice and assure her that she is familiar with her case. An alert then blinks on Dr. Tech-Savvy's screen, indicating that Ann is ready and seated in Exam Room 5.

As Dr. Tech-Savvy enters the room with a greeting and a smile, she asks Ann how she likes the practice. Ann tells her that she's very impressed. She notes that Dr. Tech-Savvy swiped a card down the side of the computer and her records magically appeared. The doctor states that she has had her staff add some basic historical information to Ann's chart so she could monitor and watch her health status over a period of time. She assures Ann that they scanned pertinent information into the system and the remainder will be maintained in paper records for the required seven years.

First, Dr. Tech-Savvy reviews her history and body systems information, which Ann had entered at home, clarifying any areas of concern. Next, she shows Ann her vital signs in a line-graph and notes that her blood pressure has gradually increased each year for the past five years. Although still within normal limits, it is something that should be monitored. Dr. Tech-Savvy then shows her a graph of her chemistry levels, which shows that her cholesterol was on the same trajectory as her blood pressure. This visual presentation makes a big impact on Ann. She had never really paid attention to the relationship between her values from year to year since they all fell into the normal or high-normal range.

Dr. Tech-Savvy clicks on a list of patient education materials and identifies those pertinent to blood pressure and cholesterol. She prints them off and sets them aside to give to Ann at the end of the visit.

Gayle appears again in the room and sits at the computer as Dr. Tech-Savvy begins Ann's physical exam. As she examines each system, Gayle annotates the doctor's findings. When the exam ends, Gayle leaves the room to greet the next patient and Dr. Tech-Savvy takes a seat in the chair facing Ann so she can add data to the computer and simultaneously review findings and a treatment plan with Ann.

While they are still together, Dr. Tech-Savvy and Ann establish a collaborative plan of care. She orders necessary tests, refills the appropriate medications from Ann's pharmacy of choice, and prints off the visit summary, which included her plan of care, vital sign and chemistry graphs, next appointment and websites available for more information, if Ann should choose to look for additional resources.

As Dr. Tech-Savvy orders a new medication for Ann's new problem, she receives a warning that Ann is allergic to that medication. So, with the click of a mouse, Dr. Tech-Savvy accesses information on another medication. As she orders the new medication, an alert appears confirming the new medication as "approved" from Ann's insurance formulary list. She finalizes the prescription order by submitting it to Ann's preferred pharmacy and prints off the patient education information on the new medication.

She ends the visit and the charge screen appears. It notes that Ann has already paid her co-pay and that her insurance will cover the remainder of the exam fee. It also asks Dr. Tech-Savvy to verify her coding, which the system extrapolated from her, and Gayle's, earlier documentation. She agrees with the findings and off goes the charge to the insurance company.

Dr. Tech-Savvy thanks Ann for coming in and lets her know she will e-mail her tomorrow regarding today's test results. She says she would like to see Ann back in one year unless she experiences any problems and to schedule any appointments from home. She reminds Ann that Gayle will return to the room to draw her blood (she no longer needs to go to the lab), and then she can leave – and to remember the information she printed off for her.

As Dr. Tech-Savvy ordered the lab work, Gayle received a message on her computer screen. Because each staff person signs in with a unique password, messages find them wherever they are working. As soon as she completed rooming Mr. Mind, she returns to Ann's room and draws her blood. Ann then dresses and heads for the pharmacy.

No need to stop and check out (where she always had to explain her story one more time), no need to make a follow-up appointment (she could do it herself!). She was done before she would've been seen by Dr. Frazzle. Ann feels empowered with information. This is – by far – her best experience with a medical group yet.

On the way home, Ann stops at her neighborhood pharmacy's drive-up window and the pharmacist hands her the medications Dr. Tech-Savvy had ordered. There is no wait because the prescriptions had been electronically sent (and were therefore legible!) while Ann was still at Tech-Savvy's office. The pharmacist explains how to take the new medication and Ann heads back to her office. Ann is no longer worried that she might forget what they told her because Dr. Tech-Savvy not only gave her written information on the new medication but also website addresses where she can learn more about her illness and the new medication.

Dr. Tech-Savvy completes her morning clinic appointments and heads to the hospital with her pocket computer. As she makes rounds, she inputs the charges so when she returns to the office she can download the charges into the system.

Today is Dr. Tech-Savvy's afternoon to spend with her family since she goes on call starting at 7 p.m. She heads home knowing that her work is complete and all the applicable charges are processed. In the old system, this would have been her afternoon to catch up. However, with the new real-time work system, she leaves with the peace of mind that nothing will fall through the cracks. Why? She did it herself and knows it is done — and the bonus is that it took less time than the traditional visit.

At 2 a.m., Dr. Tech-Savvy receives a call from the answering service that one of her partner's patients, Mr. Mind, needs medical advice and attention. She goes to her den, turns on the home computer and accesses her practice's system via a secure set of passwords. She retrieves the patient's records. She calls the patient and while speaking to him, Dr. Tech-Savvy reassures him that she is familiar with his case as well as the changes that occurred in his medication (she can see what her partner had ordered earlier in the day and automatically sent the prescription to his pharmacy of choice). She also feels that she should see him first thing in the morning, so she opens the practice schedule and with a click of the mouse schedules the appointment. There is no worry that she might forget to make a note to the patient's file or update the partner or staff about the late-night phone call. It's all in the EHR.

After getting a restful night's sleep (minus the time to answer Mr. Mind's phone call), Dr. Tech-Savvy starts her day at 6 a.m. Her first stop is her computer where she accesses the homepage and sees the results of the tests she ordered yesterday, as well as the status of the tests that are not yet finished. (This is reassuring because she no longer worries about missing test results.) As she reviews results, she checks patients' records (as needed), automatically sends notes to patients along with their results and with another click of the mouse has all the information added to the patients' EHRs.

It is now 7 a.m. and all her messages and test-result reviews are completed. She can have breakfast with her family and still get to the hospital in time for rounds before clinic starts.

As Ann goes to her computer to check her messages that same morning, she notes an e-mail from Dr. Tech-Savvy. Her lab results were fine and again Dr. Tech-Savvy has thanked her for being a patient.

Not only has EHR allowed Dr. Tech-Savvy to retain control of her practice and personal life, it made her more productive at work, eliminated most of her rework and offline work. She is able to complete today's work today. No longer does Dr. Tech-Savvy depend on others to retrieve, send or interpret messages correctly, find places to put patients in the schedule, or search for misplaced medical information or records. Records are always available and always current.

To summarize this scenario, the major advantage of the EHR is threefold:

1. Patients are empowered to take responsibility for their health. They are assured of being seen when they want to be seen and by the provider of choice with timely follow-up.

2. Physicians take back control of their practice. They now have the appropriate information at the appropriate time to see the appropriate patient and give the appropriate care.

3. Reimbursements improve. Appropriate patients with appropriate insurance and appropriate coding and timely billing result in better reimbursement in shorter time.

CHAPTER 15 | # Tying It All Together

AFTER READING THIS BOOK, you now know the basics of building an efficient and effective practice whether using a manual system or an EHR. These 7 Guiding Principles of practice management will lead to an environment where patients are happy, because meeting their needs is the cornerstone of every activity.

Staff members will see a shift in their responsibilities; however, they will enjoy stability, order, structure and freedom from "fighting fires." Physician time will be used wisely.

Do you remember the various elements of the efficient practice? Here is a quick review of the fundamentals. Do not just re-read them; think of how you can apply them.

Customer service

Build an efficient practice around patient needs. Convenient hours, courteous service, thorough explanation of tests, timely follow-up, respectful confidentiality and being proactive guardians of each patient's health and well-being all reflect positive customer service.

Let your patients be partners in their care. Moving to an EHR allows patients to take an active role in their appointments, medication, education and health status improvement.

Barrier-free practices

The efficient practice is barrier free. In a literal sense, that means that frosted glass windows do not separate the receptionist staff from the waiting room (many frosted-glass partitions are still seen today in Eastern European physician offices and connote an unfriendly, behind-the-times practice). Maybe you don't even have a waiting room. You 'greet' patients — you do not 'arrive' patients.

Efficiency extends to removing other barriers for patients. When the patient needs help, access to help is available, and help does not always have to be a physician. It means supplying information when the patient needs it and having adequate backup so a patient feels cared for at all times. The web becomes a tool for patients to access healthcare information without needing resource time from the office.

Patients schedule their own appointments

In efficient practices, deciding how much time to book for an appointment is not a matter of guesswork. Instead, specific appointment lengths and types emerge from a series of carefully crafted triage questions. This helps assure that the time booked for a patient will be long enough to meet the patient's needs without leaving the patient or physician feeling rushed. However, it is equally important that the time is not so long that you waste valuable physician time. If rules work for staff to schedule patients, they can also work for patients scheduling their own appointments.

Real-time work eliminates rework

One of the major tenets of an efficient practice is learning to do real-time work. Complete each task that you begin, do not put off work to do later. Do today's work today.

Another way of saying this is, "Do it right the first time." This is important throughout the entire practice, but the attention to detail starts at the beginning of the practice. The advantage of using an EHR is that it inherently avoids rework. Make sure your system is dynamic enough that you enter information only once and that it is accessible when needed at all levels of the system. Collect complete and accurate information. Who better to enter accurate patient information than the patient? Why have several different people interpret the same information? Handoffs are often the cause of errors. For example, a scheduler thought she heard the patient say something or it looked like the patient wrote this when it was really that. Starting out with accurate information builds credibility for the practice, shows patients a genuine concern and prevents the need to correct needless mistakes in the future.

Help physicians be productive

Policies and structure should help doctors work smarter, not harder. To do this, physicians should perform tasks that only they can do safely. If you can safely and legally delegate downward, do it.

Staff members can do many tasks to save physician time: identify a patient's chief complaint, take vital signs, stock exam rooms appropriately, and so on.

These steps mean that the physician can walk into the exam room, greet the patient by name, focus on the presenting complaint, complete the exam, develop the treatment plan, complete the order sheet and provide resource materials without scurrying around.

The physician is not distracted with needless details, so s/he can provide the single most important patient criterion for a good visit, "The doctor really listened to me."

The EHR allows the physician to complete his/her work while in the exam room. This is real-time work at its best.

Hold a morning huddle

The entire staff should meet for a few minutes every day. The daily agenda is simple and includes three items:

1. Is there any follow-up work from yesterday that needs to be completed?

2. Are there any anticipated problems or challenges in today's schedule?

3. Are there any problems with tomorrow's schedule that we can address today?

This daily meeting is a great way to quickly share information with the entire staff, thank people for extra effort, answer questions and address concerns.

Make communication routine and painless

Every day physicians and staff must process dozens of items of information. Good systems can make this happen efficiently. Evaluate the speed of response, the best person to respond and use the systems outlined in this book.

The underlying concepts

Years of experience go into building an efficient practice, as well as several key concepts, which are worth remembering. The next few paragraphs explain the concepts that are the underpinning of all efficient practices.

Decisions made from data always are better than actions based on hunches. One piece of information does not establish a trend. One fact is not all you need to know; nor is one anecdote the whole story.

Those professionals running the most successful practices today make decisions based on solid information, collected over time, analyzed carefully and responded to with well-crafted solutions.

If you want to know what your customers want, ask them. Put patients in charge of the practice. Ask them what they want. Develop a website that allows patients to ask questions, get information and schedule their own appointments. Don't forget to include a survey – you need to better understand your patients' needs.

If you ask them, patients will be your strongest allies in building a practice that genuinely meets their needs. More important, if you listen and act on what a patient tells you, you will build loyalty that will last a lifetime.

Make all office functions support the core practice. At its core, a medical practice is about a physician spending time with a patient. Aim every activity and process at making that encounter go smoothly, easily and successfully for both the physician and the patient.

If you peel off the many layers of a practice, this is the pearl that you will find at the center – physicians who enjoy seeing patients.

Take the team approach. It is not good use of a physician's time to stock exam rooms. Similarly, it does not make sense for a receptionist to give medical advice. Remember to delegate tasks to the lowest-skill-level person who can do the task safely, legally and with credibility.

Efficient practices give great customer service. From the first encounter with an efficiently and effectively run practice, it is immediately apparent that the practice values customer service. The staff quickly responds to people by name, listens attentively, responds with concern and strives to accommodate their wishes.

A new patient will experience that sense of service throughout his or her visit. Wait times will be minimal. The physician will spend focused time with the patient by being attentive and informative. Follow-up communication will be timely, understandable and warm.

In an efficient practice, you treat every patient like a first-class honored customer.

Make things uniform; strive for standardization. The physicians in a practice should decide what protocols, standards, vendors and supplies they want to use and stick to those decisions. Variation creates waste. The need for more money in inventory, duplicate training and systems that may not be integrated is costly. The more variation there is, the less support physicians feel. Variation creates complex systems that result in increased errors, inefficiencies and rework.

If there is only one physician, obviously there is only one standard. When two physicians work together, it becomes more complex. When you have 10 or more physicians in a practice, variations for each of them can cause absolute chaos. One practice cut the costs of cataract surgery by 40 percent simply by agreeing to use the same supplies and negotiating a good price from the supplier. The rule: establish one way of doing things and stick to it unless the group decides to change.

When these principles are put into place, a practice invariably runs more smoothly, increases patient satisfaction, leads to more productive, happy physicians and staff, and adds to the practice's profitability.

We've illustrated how the EHR allows for real-time work, eliminates non-value-added labor costs and allows patients to work with you. There are many EHR vendors; shop around. As you consider implementing such a system in your practice, consider these features:

- ■ Relational database – only enter information once;
- ■ Interactive website;
- ■ Internal and external email access;
- ■ Digital picture and personal information;
- ■ Summary page;
- ■ Remote access;
- ■ Alerts;
- ■ Notes to queue activities;
- ■ Pharmacy module with formulary information;

- Order entry system including test verification and results reporting;

- Coding from documentation;

- Voice recognition;

- Data search capability;

- Patient visit summary;

- Patient appointment scheduling;

- Access to patient education material;

- Access to medical information;

- Practice management system, EHR and scheduling system integration;

- Connectivity to payers;

- Easy navigation; and

- Time-stamped activities for workflow analysis.

We encourage you to put these recommendations to the test in your own organization and embrace the 7 Guiding Principles of Medical Practice Management with EHR technology. The results will delight you and your patients.

Glossary

Ambulatory practice – A practice that provides outpatient, non-hospitalized services, such as diagnosis, treatment, outpatient surgery and rehabilitation.

Barrier-free practice – The barrier-free practice has removed figurative and literal obstacles, such as sliding reception windows, and provides computer access to create a patient-focused practice.

Call schedule – The schedule that shows when each physician is on call for a practice.

Charge capture – The opportunity to note charges for each procedure, visit or other provider charges for inpatient and outpatient care on the patient's bill.

Demographic history – Patient information that includes name, address, telephone, insurance, etc.

Discharge – Preparing a patient to leave the office visit by providing information the patient needs for health education, test preparation, etc.

Documentation – The physician's notes regarding the patient's diagnosis and treatment, and applicable billing codes.

Efficient practice – A practice that uses the seven practice-management guidelines to work together in a seamless process of patient care.

Electronic health record – An EHR is a computer system that contains and maintains patient information and allows patient and provider access to that system.

Electronic signature – A digital or computerized signature.

Encounter – A patient's office visit, defined by MGMA as "a documented, face-to-face contact between a patient and a provider who exercises independent judgment in the provision of services to the individual in an ambulatory or hospital setting." (Data such as diagnosis and services provided are included on the patient's bill.)

Episodic care – A chronological list of a patient's health history and medical care.

HIPAA – The Health Insurance Portability and Accountability Act of 1996, which protects health insurance coverage for workers and their families when they change or lose their jobs.

Licensed practical nurse (LPN) – An LPN is a graduate of an accredited nursing school who passed the state board of nursing exam. LPNs must be re-licensed biannually. The LPN scope of function differs from state to state. Generally, LPNs work under the direction of a doctor or registered nurse and perform the same health care services as a medical assistant plus these additional tasks: receive verbal orders from the physician; administer drugs; medications; treatment; tests; injections; inoculations and blood or blood products; review lab results; and initiate, monitor and regulate peripheral IV therapy. An LPN may also provide telephone or in-person patient education with physician direction.

Medical assistant – Each state dictates the scope of the MA position. Usually MAs may provide administrative, clerical and technical support for physicians. They must receive certification to take X-rays and perform venipunctures and other procedures. Depending on state regulations, MAs may: take routine vitals; determine reason for visit; assess for pain, abuse, nutritional and functional needs, and learning barriers; ensure supplies are available; set up sterile field for procedures; complete medication list and document allergies; ensure medical record is complete; make follow-up appointments; maintain tickler file for abnormal test results; begin referral process; verify and report lab results.

Mid-level provider – See Nonphysician provider.

Mission statement – A written statement that describes the purpose and vision or goal for your practice.

Nonphysician provider — Nonphysician providers can be nurse practitioners or physician assistants. They are licensed by each state and nationally certified to work under a physician's direction in diagnosing and treating patients as well as prescriptive privileges.

Offline work – When a practice is inefficient, it does not complete tasks at the time they present. Offline work includes returning messages, dictation and billing.

Online work – An efficient practice completes all tasks or work as they present.

Scheduling outliers – Issues that are barriers to scheduling patients for appropriate exam times, such as: patient on multiple medicines, patient seen by multiple physicians over the past year, or a new patient with a complicated medical history.

Open-access scheduling – A system of patient scheduling that allows patients to be seen when they want to be seen by provider of choice.

Operational system – The systems in place that run a practice: how phones are answered, how patients are scheduled, how payments are collected, how patient education and communications are handled.

Outcome – The results of a patient's course of treatment.

Out-of-pocket charges – Charges that are not paid by a health insurance company or health plan, but that are paid by a patient.

Patient compliance – When a patient complies with your treatment and education protocols.

Patient-focused setting – A practice that caters to patient cares and needs.

Physician productivity – Seeing the appropriate number of patients daily while completing all work in real time.

Protected e-mail – Electronic mail that is protected from viruses and junk mail and maintains confidentiality.

Protocol – Guidelines for handling treatments and medical advice.

Real-time work – Completing work at the time the work appears, not leaving it for later.

Registered nurse – A graduate from a formal nursing education program who holds a current state nursing license. RNs must have substantial specialized knowledge, judgment and skill based on the principles of biological, physiological, behavioral and sociological science. Depending on state regulations, they may perform all MA and LPN tasks and are accountable for all nursing practice including: observation; assessment; care or counsel; health teaching; and health maintenance and prevention. At the direction of a provider, RNs may administer treatments; tests; medications; IV therapies and inoculations and routine vision screenings. They supervise the front office staff, MAs and LPNs.

Revenue generating activities – A practice generates revenue by seeing patients both in the office and in the hospital.

Scheduling rules – These rules govern how patients are scheduled. They may include: length of time for short, medium and long visits, number of physicians in the office every day, and the reason for the visit as it relates to the length of visit.

Practice standardization – Areas in practice systems in which consistency increases efficiency and decreases costs, such as: medical supply vendors.

Tech-savvy – A person who is up-to-date on technology and uses it to improve efficiency.

Variation in a practice – Multiple ways of handling practice systems.

Voice-recognition software – A software computer program that recognizes voices and types what the voice says.

Workflow – The steps in a business process; tasks that need to be done and the order in which they need to be completed.

Index

Access, ix, 1, 3, 23, 26, 40, 55, 62, 73, 95-96, 104, 108-109, 111, 113
Accounting, 97
Action box, 62, 91-92
Administrators, 82-83
Ambulatory practice, 68, 111
Appointment type, 54, 77, 79
Appointments, 19, 23, 26, 30, 40, 46, 50-51, 54, 56, 63-64, 69, 71, 90, 100, 104, 107, 112
  patient-scheduled, 104
ASAP, 60-62, 64, 91

Billing, 13, 24, 27-28, 29, 60, 63-64, 69, 87, 92, 102, 111-112, 113
Bottlenecks, 40
Brainstorming, 51
Business administration, 27

Call schedule, 34, 47, 111
Change, ix, 3, 6, 14, 20, 30, 40, 50-51, 82, 91, 97, 108, 112
Charge capture, 13, 111
Charges, out-of-pocket, 27, 113
Clinic days, 33
Coding, 60, 72, 99, 102, 109
Communication, 1-2, 13-14, 22-23, 26, 27, 44, 64, 76-77, 79-80, 81-83, 87, 95, 106-107
Continuous stopwatch time study, 36
Core practice, 2, 107
Customer service, 5, 17, 27, 62, 103, 107

Data, 42, 53, 99, 106, 109, 112
Database, 53, 108
Delays, 24, 62, 63
Delegation, 14, 73, 105, 107
Demographic history, 111

Dictation, 13, 36, 38, 60, 79, 91, 113
Documentation, 3, 30, 60, 64, 87, 92, 99, 109, 111
Dollars-per-visit, 34, 39
Duties, statement of, 67, 69-70

Efficient practice, x, 2-3, 15, 61, 65, 75, 92, 103-104, 106-107, 111, 113
Electronic health records (EHR), 1, 3, 25, 26, 30, 42, 51, 56, 57, 59, 60, 63, 64, 77, 79, 80, 87, 93, 95, 97, 101-105, 108, 109, 111
  benefits of, 25-26, 28, 63, 102
Electronic signature, 112
Employee, performance evaluation, 71
Episodic care, 112
Evaluation, 53, 71
Exam room, 6-7, 14, 22, 24-25, 30, 37-38, 42, 44, 56, 72, 77-78, 85-87, 90-92, 96-98, 105
  stocking, 71, 90
Follow-up, 6, 26, 30, 46, 50, 53, 59, 63-64, 68, 79-81, 90, 92, 100, 102-103, 106-107, 112

Guiding Principles, x, 30, 109
  7 Guiding Principles of Medical Practice Management, 12-15, 109
  Principle I, 12, 29; II, 13, 31; III, 13, 43; IV, 14, 49, 76; V, 14, 67; VI, 14, 75; VII, 14, 85

Health Insurance Portability and Accountability Act (HIPAA), 95, 112
Housekeeping, 65

In box, 6, 9, 61, 62
Interdependent team, 12, 14, 75-76

Job description, 70-71

Mail, 62
Medical
   assistant, 23, 70, 74, 112
   records department, 89
Medical Group Management
   Association (MGMA), ix, 112
Mission statement, 15, 17-21, 76, 83,
   112

Nonphysician providers, 46, 74, 85,
   113
Nurses
   Registered (RN), 23, 62, 65, 68, 70,
     72-73, 89, 112, 114
   Licensed Practical (LPN), 68, 73,
     112, 114

Office, ix-x, 6-9, 13, 15, 19, 22-24, 26-
   29, 32-35, 54, 57, 59, 68-69, 71,
   73, 75-77, 85, 87, 89-92, 96, 100,
   104, 107, 111-112, 114
Operational system, 113
Out box, 61-62, 91, 92
Outliers, 51, 54, 112, 113

Paperwork, 2, 4, 60, 61
Patient, x, 19, 55, 89
   compliance, 14, 113
   discharge, 59, 111
   expectations, 1, 14, 21-22
   throughput, 40-41, 42
Patient visit order sheet, 79-81
Patient visit worksheet, 78-79
Phones, 63
Physician, 2-3, 5, 9, 11, 13-15, 17-18,
   25-26, 28, 32-34, 36-40, 43, 45-
   46, 49-52, 54-56, 59, 61-64, 67,
   72-74, 76, 79, 81-83, 85, 95-96,
   98, 102, 105-108, 112-114
   compensation, 34-35
   productivity, 105
Practices, ix, 3, 5, 11-12, 15, 17-18,
   21, 32, 39-40, 43-44, 46, 49, 51,
   53, 72, 85-86, 104, 106-107
   barrier-free, 104, 111
   proactive, 11
Productivity, 5, 32, 39, 47, 50, 55, 62,
   73, 82, 85, 113
Protocols, 2, 57, 65, 73, 108, 113
Real-time work, x, 9, 12, 29-31, 101,
   104-105, 108, 114

Records, 3, 25, 36, 53, 56, 69, 72, 78,
   80, 89, 91, 95-98, 101-102
Reimbursement, 28, 102
Remarks, 53, 77-78
Resource allocation, x, 12, 14-15, 84,
   85-87
Revenue, ix, 34, 38-39, 114
Review, 7, 20, 36, 38, 53, 56, 59-60,
   71-72, 79, 81-82, 90-91, 95, 97,
   99, 103, 112
Rooming, 57-59, 64, 68-69, 79, 100

Schedule, 1, 6, 13, 23, 27, 30, 32-34,
   36, 39-40, 43-47, 50-51, 54-56,
   62, 64, 74, 77, 81-82, 89-91, 96,
   98, 100-102, 104, 106-107, 111
   balanced master, 45-46
Scheduling, 23
   open-access, 55
   outliers, 113
   rules, 50-54
Self-analysis tool, 37-38
Staff, ix, 2-3, 5, 7, 11-15, 17-18, 20,
   22-24, 26-28, 31, 36, 39-40, 42-
   45, 47, 50-51, 54-64, 67-68, 71-
   83, 85-86, 90, 98, 100-101, 103-
   108, 114
   suppport, 39, 43, 52
Standardization, 14, 108, 114
State Board of Medicine, 74
Stock, 7, 56-57, 105, 107
Systems, ix-x, 1-2, 5, 9, 12, 21-22, 28,
   49-50, 55, 59, 63-65, 75-76, 79,
   93, 95, 98, 106, 108, 113-114

Task distribution, 12, 67, 69-70, 72-
   74, 76, 104, 106
Teams, 14, 76, 83
Teamwork, 9, 11-12, 14, 74-75, 81-82
Time inventory, 39
Tracking, 40, 64
Training, 57, 73, 108
Triage, 14, 54, 61, 65, 68, 72-73, 104

Variation, decreasing unnecessary, x,
   12, 14, 49-65, 76
Voice-recognition, 114

Waiting area, 24
Work
   offline, 13, 102, 113
   online, 113
   volume of, 12-14, 69, 71, 83, 85-86
Workflow, 5, 61, 109, 114
Workloads, 39, 47
   balancing, 13, 43